Bariatric Slow Cooker Cookbook

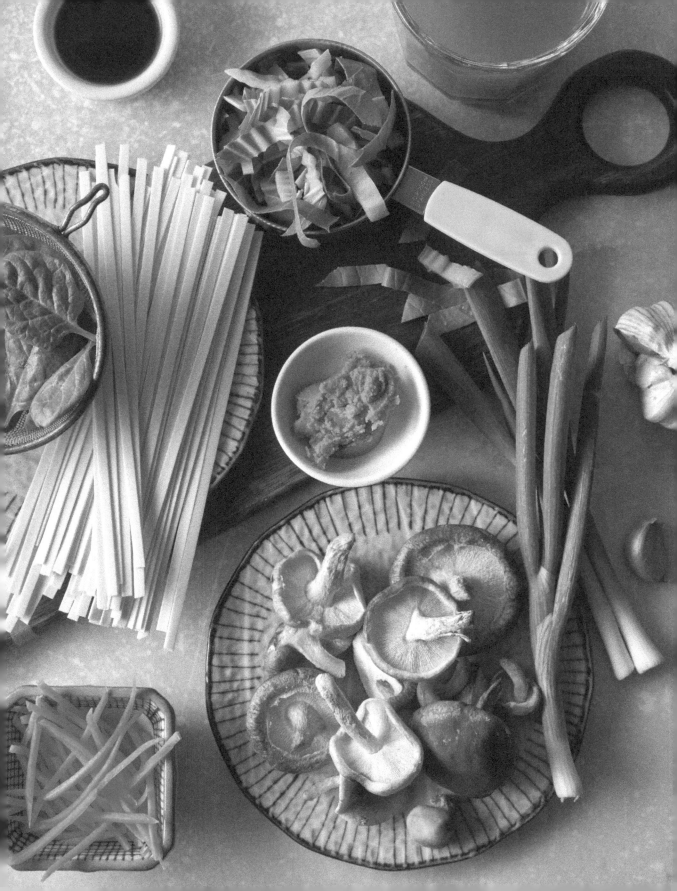

BARIATRIC
slow *cooker*
COOKBOOK

Easy Recipes for Post-Op Recovery and Lifelong Health

Lauren Minchen, MPH, RDN, CDN

Photography by Darren Muir

ROCKRIDGE PRESS

For general information on our other products and services or to obtain technical support, please contact our Customer Care Department within the United States at (866) 744-2665, or outside the United States at (510) 253-0500.

Rockridge Press publishes its books in a variety of electronic and print formats. Some content that appears in print may not be available in electronic books, and vice versa.

TRADEMARKS: Rockridge Press and the Rockridge Press logo are trademarks or registered trademarks of Callisto Media Inc. and/or its affiliates, in the United States and other countries, and may not be used without written permission. All other trademarks are the property of their respective owners. Rockridge Press is not associated with any product or vendor mentioned in this book.

Interior and Cover Designer: Darren Samuel
Art Producer: Maya Melenchuk
Editor: Marjorie DeWitt
Production Editor: Ashley Polikoff

Cover: Very Veggie Lasagna, page 92
Photography © 2022 Darren Muir

Paperback ISBN: 978-1-638-07313-0
eBook ISBN: 978-1-638-07217-1
R0

CONTENTS

INTRODUCTION

Are you recently recovering from bariatric surgery? Is your bariatric procedure in the near future? Are you wondering how you'll get through your recovery while also adjusting to a new way of eating? If you answered yes to any of these questions, you're in the right place! Bariatric surgery brings with it many physical, psychological, and emotional changes that relate to your lifestyle and eating habits, but preparing safe and healthy food after bariatric surgery doesn't have to be difficult. Although it can feel incredibly daunting, I'm here to show you that developing a new eating plan that prioritizes your health and healing can be easy and that you can achieve your goals while enjoying the process along the way.

I am a Registered Dietitian Nutritionist, and I have been working in the nutrition field for about 10 years. I work with many bariatric surgery clients who are at a loss as to how to approach their new way of life. They may feel fearful of the unknown and unsure of how to navigate their new normal while also managing the pressure they feel to see results. Making these big adjustments as easy as possible is essential to helping them build lifelong healthy habits. I work with them to find meals they love, identify foods they don't like so much, determine the time and energy they have for meal prep and then develop a personalized plan that empowers them to create and sustain healthy habits. And that's why I am creating these recipes for you here.

Your journey toward success postsurgery should be a process that, although challenging and new, is something you can enjoy and build upon. Postsurgery, you can look forward to doing more things that you love. Maybe you want to pick up a sport or hobby you haven't been able to before now. Or maybe you simply want to travel more comfortably. Establishing a better food routine that you can rely upon is also something you can look forward to after you've recovered and become familiar with your new eating pattern. A food routine can help reduce anxiety around food choices, promote consistent digestion, and create stability around meals and snacks. Both being able to do things you love and establishing a food routine are part of the total improvement in your overall quality of life after surgery. And the healthy habits you build now will be the things that help you achieve and maintain these goals.

As you are adjusting to a new way of life, slow-cooking allows you to maximize your nutrition through protein-rich foods and makes prepping meals easy. Especially during recovery when you need rest, easy options with minimal steps will be key. Keeping things easy is also the best way to begin to build healthy habits. The slow cooker is a valuable tool to use during your healing and recovery. I hope you enjoy these recipes and the process as you learn the ropes of your slow cooker!

Although this book won't cover your recovery in its entirety, it will provide you with some helpful tips and recipes that will make your recovery and lifelong health goals easier to achieve—and enjoyable. So, browse the recipes, become familiar with those that are best for various stages of your recovery, and get ready to do some slow-cooking! I hope you enjoy making these as much as I enjoyed creating them for you.

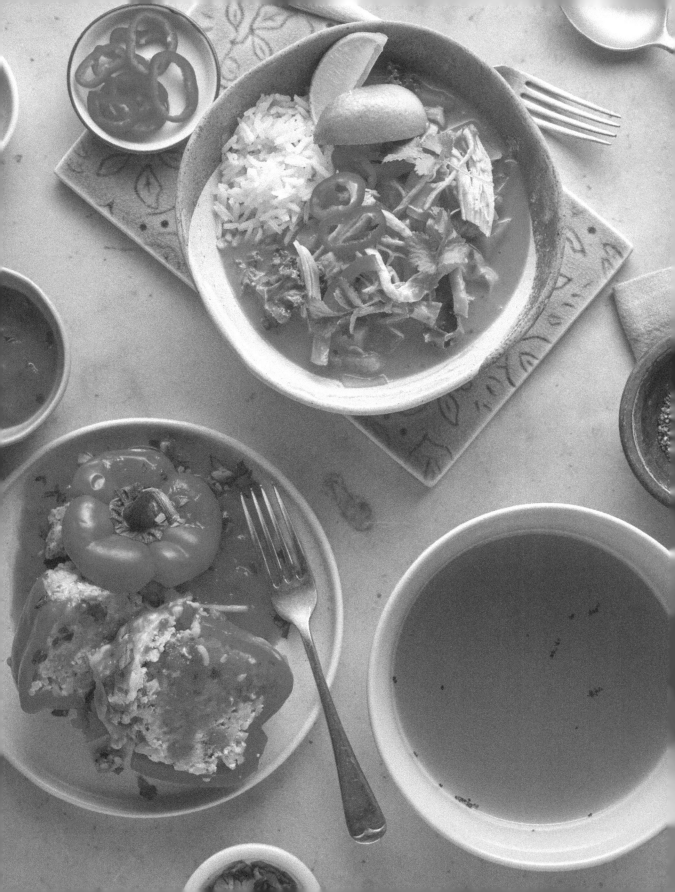

1
Slow & Steady

Are you ready to dive into some seriously easy meals? Maybe you recently made it through bariatric surgery, or maybe your surgery is coming up soon. Either way, you're probably wondering what and how to eat during your recovery. Look no further! This cookbook will provide you with staples, comforting favorites, and unique creations—all that support your healing and recovery while requiring minimal effort and prep.

Healing with Your Slow Cooker

Many, if not most, of my bariatric clients assume that building healthy eating habits after surgery means committing to hours of work in the kitchen. I quickly reassure them that this could not be further from the truth! During recovery, it's important to have quick and easy recipes that allow time for rest and healing.

Using a slow cooker is a great way to minimize your time in the kitchen. Although cooking times can be longer than cooking in the oven or on the stovetop, the number of steps you need to follow and the time spent supervising the process are greatly reduced. Often, you can simply put all of the ingredients into the slow cooker and step away until it's done. This saved prep time and effort is essential when you are recovering from surgery.

Incorporating the use of your slow cooker into your weekly routine can also boost your intake of fiber- and vitamin-rich vegetables, legumes, and whole grains that you may otherwise not have time to prepare for yourself. After surgery and during recovery, your top nutritional needs include protein, fiber, vitamin B12, folate, iron, vitamin D, and calcium. Consuming natural foods rich in these vitamins and minerals is essential for energy, recovery, and a healthy digestive system. Building appropriate eating habits that meet your postsurgery needs takes time, but making this process as easy as possible means that you are more likely to commit to the changes and maintain them over time.

In this book, I will provide you with a variety of slow cooker recipes that are rich in essential nutrients and also easy to digest. I've included plant-based recipes, meat and poultry dishes, and nourishing desserts so you have a range of choices for nutritious dishes that will satisfy whatever you may be craving. Have fun with the recipes. Find your favorites. And most of all, enjoy the convenience as you nourish yourself, rest, and recover.

Hidden Health Benefits of Slow-Cooking

Your slow cooker is an easy way to prepare protein-rich meals. But that's not the only thing it's good for! Here are several more benefits of using your slow cooker:

Greater food variety. Because of its ability to boost flavor naturally while keeping prep simple, slow-cooking may help diversify the nutritious foods you consume and, as a result, improve your intake of a variety of essential nutrients.

Flavorful healthy foods. Healthy doesn't have to mean bland! Slow-cooking allows any added spices, herbs, and liquids to develop a richer flavor and texture than with traditional stovetop or oven cooking, particularly because of the reduced temperature and extended cooking time.

Lower and healthier fat content. The slow-cooking process gives you control over the amount of oil you use in your meals, and it also means consumption of fewer processed foods that are high in fat.

Preserved nutrient profile of foods. Because of the slow cooker's lower cooking temperature, vitamins, minerals, and phytonutrients are more readily preserved, helping you optimize your essential nutrient intake during your healing and recovery.

Reduced sodium intake. With the use of a variety of herbs and spices, as well as the natural rich flavors from various meats and plant foods at your disposal, you can easily reduce sodium without losing flavor and richness in your meals.

Post-Op Recovery

Postoperation, the consistency of your food will be regulated over the course of your recovery period, progressing from clear liquids to liquids and then pureed foods, followed by soft foods and finally to a general diet. This section shows you how you can use your slow cooker at each of these stages. Your specific diet progression will be determined by your bariatric team, but the following timelines reflect a typical schedule.

LAPBAND AND GASTRIC SLEEVE

FIRST 1–2 DAYS	CLEAR LIQUIDS
WEEKS 1–2	LIQUIDS
WEEK 3	PUREED FOODS
WEEKS 4–6	SOFT FOODS
WEEKS 7–8+	GENERAL DIET

What to Avoid

To prevent discomfort or irritation, do your best to avoid the following foods for at least three months after your surgery:

› Alcohol

› Caffeine

› Carbonated beverages (seltzer, soda, kombucha)

› Crunchy foods, like chips, pretzels, and raw vegetables

- Dried fruits, like raisins, dried cranberries, and apricots
- Dry foods, like nuts, granola, and dry cereals
- Greasy, oily, and fried foods
- Heavily spiced foods
- Microwaved foods, due to the removal of moisture
- Sugar alcohols (erythritol, maltitol, glycerol, mannitol, sorbitol, xylitol)
- Sugary drinks
- Tough or dry red meat

If you experience any pain, nausea, vomiting, dizziness, sweating, or diarrhea after eating, something you ate may not be sitting well with you. If you still experience persistent symptoms after eliminating bothersome foods, consult with your doctor.

Liquids

During this initial post-op stage, you will want to consume between 48 and 64 ounces of fluid per day, ideally broken up into five or six liquid meals. For some, the liquids stage may be divided into two stages: clear liquids and all liquids. During the clear liquids phase, stick to broth, water, 2 percent milk, or gelatin. During the second liquids phase, you may be able to include some thicker liquids, like vegetable soups.

SLOW COOKER STANDOUTS:

Savory Chicken Broth (clear liquids) (page 144)

Savory Vegetable Broth (clear liquids) (page 146)

Butternut Squash Soup (second liquids phase) (page 63)

PRE-OP PREP:

You will feel weak and tired the first two weeks after surgery, so this is the most important stage to prep ahead for. Before surgery, make a batch of each of the broths and freeze them.

Pureed Foods

During this stage, you will aim to consume three meals per day, focusing mostly on protein-rich pureed foods, like plain or blended yogurt (no fruit chunks), cream-based soups (no vegetable chunks), mashed cottage cheese (small curd), scrambled eggs, mashed white fish, canned mashed chicken breast, mashed root vegetables, oatmeal, pureed fruits, and pureed vegetables. These foods should be free of chunks and mashed or pureed until smooth and creamy in texture.

SLOW COOKER STANDOUTS:

Creamy Homemade Greek Yogurt (page 90)

No-Sugar-Added Applesauce (page 138)

Tuscan Chicken and White Bean Stew (page 59)

Savory Mashed Root Vegetables (page 45)

PRE-OP PREP:

You may be feeling slightly more energetic as you graduate to this stage of your recovery. However, your stomach will still be unable to break down any food that is not pureed. Before surgery, cook one batch each of the Creamy Homemade Greek Yogurt (page 90) and No-Sugar-Added Applesauce (page 138) and freeze them. Each of these will keep for an additional two weeks once you move them to the refrigerator. The Tuscan Chicken and White Bean Stew (page 59) and Savory Mashed Root Vegetables (page 45) will need to be prepared the week that you move into this phase. Each will last for one week in the refrigerator.

Soft Foods

During the soft-foods stage, you will aim to consume three meals per day, focusing on protein-rich foods like chicken, fish, and soft meats. You will also include cottage cheese, yogurt, cooked vegetables, soft fruits, cooked cereals like oatmeal, and legumes. Avoid seeds and uncooked skins on fruits and vegetables. Drink 48 to 64 ounces of fluid (water and sugar-free drinks) per day, and try to drink most of this between meals.

SLOW COOKER STANDOUTS:

Shakshuka (page 30)

Cheesy Cauliflower, Broccoli, and Carrots (page 50)

Easy Chicken and Rice (page 98)

Simple Ground Turkey and Vegetables (page 107)

Cinnamon Apples and Pears (page 133)

PRE-OP PREP:

Before your surgery, plan to purchase as many ingredients as you can to have on hand as you transition into this phase of recovery. If possible, try to plan your menu before surgery, and stock up on nonperishables like rice, beans, and rolled oats.

When planning your menu, follow recommended freezing times (specified at the end of each recipe). It's also helpful to freeze food in small or medium portions so you can thaw only what you need. When thawing frozen food, it's preferable to thaw it in the refrigerator overnight, then heat it on the stovetop over low heat, as needed, to thaw it completely.

General Foods

Achieving this stage in recovery means you can eat foods of normal consistency. However, the volume you are able to eat will remain smaller than it was presurgery. Aim to eat either three balanced meals or six small snack-like meals per day, depending on your

Protein: A Slow Cooker Star

During your postsurgery healing process, you will need to consume protein every time you eat, which is at least three times per day. Protein is best digested and utilized when it is consumed in moderate portions consistently throughout the day (as opposed to once per day or inadequate intake throughout the day), so focusing each meal on high-quality proteins will maximize its benefit in your recovery.

Making sure you get adequate protein in every meal can take some focus, but luckily, protein happens to be one of the things the slow cooker does best! Slow-cooking provides moist heat, which breaks up the protein's connective tissue between muscle fibers and softens it. This softening makes meats easier to chew and digest, which is particularly helpful for you during your recovery. In addition, the low heat of a slow cooker means your meal is less likely to overcook. Finally, the slow cooker makes it easy to season meat, poultry, and fish as you like them because it allows you to adjust spice intensity over a long cooking period. You can start small with seasoning and add more toward the end of the cooking time so that you achieve your desired flavor.

When looking for protein, prioritize protein-dense foods that are also lower in calories. Some heavy or greasy foods may contain a decent amount of protein, but their heaviness may prevent you from being able to eat enough to achieve the desired protein intake. You will be better able to meet your daily protein needs during this time if you focus on lean protein sources. In general, look for foods that contain 10 grams of protein per 100 calories. The higher the protein grams and the lower the calories, the easier it will be to get the protein you need each day.

Protein is important after bariatric surgery for the following reasons:

Protein assists in proper wound healing. Protein actively supports tissue repair and collagen synthesis by providing essential amino acids and minerals like zinc, iron, and copper.

Protein supports your metabolism. Protein exerts a thermic effect on the body, increasing metabolism. It also requires more energy (calories) to digest. Together, these factors can help you use more calories all day long, including while you sleep.

Protein helps you feel full longer. Protein boosts satiety (the feeling of fullness) and helps you feel satisfied after eating meals. In turn, this prevents you from feeling hungry and helps build consistent, healthy eating habits.

Protein helps form hormones, enzymes, and antibodies to help your body function properly. Consuming adequate protein supports every function of your body and is essential for hormonal health, immune health, and metabolic health.

Protein boosts your intake of essential vitamins and minerals. Lean protein foods are rich in B vitamins, zinc, iron, selenium, and magnesium, which support your immune system, energy production, metabolism, wound healing, digestion, and inflammation management.

Slow-Cooking Protein Stars

FOOD	AMOUNT	CALORIES	PROTEIN (GRAMS)
CHICKEN BREAST	1 OUNCE	50	9
TURKEY BREAST	1 OUNCE	55	5
SALMON	1 OUNCE	33	5
COD	1 OUNCE	50	5
HALIBUT	1 OUNCE	32	6
90/10 LEAN BEEF	1 OUNCE	50	6
LEAN PORK LOIN	1 OUNCE	41	6
EGG	1 WHOLE	70	6
1 PERCENT COTTAGE CHEESE	¼ CUP	40	7
FIRM TOFU	⅓ CUP	50	5

volume tolerance. Prioritize protein- and nutrient-rich foods (think fruits and vegetables), since you won't be able to eat as much in one sitting. Save fluids for between meals.

SLOW COOKER STANDOUTS:

Veggie Lover's Breakfast Casserole (page 23)

Hearty Beef and Barley Stew (page 66)

Salmon, Pasta, and Vegetable Bake (page 80)

Maple-Balsamic Lamb Shoulder (page 122)

Reduced-Sugar Chocolate–Chocolate Chip Lava Cake (page 129)

Eating Well for Life

Nourishing your body after surgery is essential for achieving and maintaining the results you are looking for. Once you've reached the general-foods stage, these principles will be essential for reaching your goals and creating lifelong healthy eating habits.

Prioritize protein at every meal. Protein supports tissue repair, collagen synthesis, fullness, metabolic health, energy, hormonal health, and immunity when consumed in adequate and consistent portions. The slow cooker is the perfect tool to make foods rich in protein, like chicken, fish, seafood, lean beef, lean pork, eggs, and tofu.

Eat foods high in fiber. Fiber is essential for managing appetite, supporting a healthy digestive tract, and stabilizing blood sugar. The slow cooker is great for cooking high-fiber foods like brown rice, quinoa, legumes, and root vegetables.

Consume a moderate amount of healthy fats. Healthy fats and oils (think wild fish, olive oil, avocado, and nut or seed butters) are essential for energy, cell health, brain health, satiety, and a healthy metabolism. The slow cooker can help boost your healthy fat intake by reducing the need to add saturated fat content to dishes.

Focus on fruits and vegetables. Fresh and frozen produce provides essential vitamins, minerals, phytonutrients, and other antioxidants that support tissue healing, collagen synthesis, immunity, healthy aging, and the prevention of chronic diseases. Slow-cooking can help make fruits and vegetables easier to consume, particularly during certain recovery phases.

Keep meals small and frequent. To maintain your success after bariatric surgery, it's essential to pace yourself regarding your food intake. Eating too much at once can cause pain, discomfort, and complications, whereas eating infrequently can lead to excessive hunger and cravings. With the slow cooker, prep is easy and you can cook in large batches, store them in the refrigerator or freezer, and reheat them as needed, so you always have healthy meals on hand.

Stay hydrated. Drinking enough water aids your recovery journey and your weight-management goals by supporting your metabolism, encouraging a healthy appetite, keeping your digestive tract smooth, and giving you energy. The slow cooker can boost your liquid consumption by making the preparation of soups and broths easy.

Chew your food thoroughly. Take some burden off your stomach by chewing thoroughly at mealtime. Swallowing large bites or chunks of poorly chewed food can place an enormous burden on your healing stomach. The slow cooker can help with this by increasing the tenderness and softening the texture of the foods you cook with it.

Minimize processed foods with little nutritional value. Prioritize nutrient-dense foods, and save high-sugar and high-fat foods for special occasions. Doing so promotes adequate nutrient consumption, supports your recovery and overall health, and helps you reach your weight-management goal. Slow-cooking can help you prioritize nourishing foods by making meal prep simple.

Portion Control

Practicing proper portion control will support your recovery and healing while helping you move toward your weight-management goal. Eating high-quality foods is important for overall health, but using proper portions is essential for healthy digestion and weight management. Each of the recipes in this book will provide stage-specific serving sizes so that you know exactly how much to serve.

Stage-by-Stage Serving Sizes

Liquids: ¼ cup–½ cup

Pureed Foods: ¼ cup–½ cup

Soft Foods: ½ cup

General Foods: ½ cup to 1 cup

Tips

› Store meals in single-serving containers.

› Serve yourself a single portion, and put the rest away.

› Keep a serving-size guide on your refrigerator or cabinet.

› Prioritize nutrient- and protein-rich foods to boost fullness.

› Don't skip meals. Make sure you have meals prepped and ready to go to stay consistent.

Golden Rules of Slow-Cooking

There are some best practices when it comes to cooking successfully with a slow cooker. Here are some golden rules of slow-cooking:

Don't open the lid. Opening the lid adds 15 minutes to the total cooking time, so avoid this until you need to gauge progress. Typically, this means waiting to check progress until there's about 30 to 45 minutes left, then extending the cooking time as needed after checking.

Layer ingredients properly. The majority of the slow cooker's heat comes from the bottom, so the toughest ingredients need to be added first (meats, root vegetables), followed by more-fragile ingredients (fruits and vegetables). Then the liquid should be poured over the top to submerge those ingredients and prevent them from drying out.

Don't add too much alcohol. For any recipe that calls for wine, beer, or spirits, watch the portions. Too much alcohol in the mix can leave a boozy flavor and aroma because it may not have enough time to boil off due to low cooking temperatures. Typically, just a splash of alcohol is enough in a slow cooker.

Practice flexibility with cooking time and temperature. Did you know that slow cookers vary when it comes to cooking time and temperature? Sometimes, a recipe may not turn out as described, and that's okay. Simply practice it with different temperatures and cooking times until you get it right for your slow cooker. For example, if you noticed that a recipe was too done when following the recommended cooking time and temperature, try reducing the cooking time by 30 minutes next time you make it. Conversely, if a recipe is undercooked, simply increase the cooking time in 30-minute increments until the desired doneness is reached. Save temperature changes (high to low or vice versa) only for when a shift in cooking time is not achieving the desired results, because a temperature shift will most likely induce a significant shift in cooking time.

Release extra liquid at the end of cooking time. If the meat is finished cooking but you still observe too much liquid, simply take off the lid of your slow cooker and increase the temperature setting to high. Let it cook 30 to 45 minutes longer so the extra liquid can boil off. This should help increase the thickness of any remaining liquid (if you're going for more of a gravy-like texture).

Fill your slow cooker appropriately. Don't overfill your slow cooker! When you do so, it causes the food to steam rather than simmer, which translates to longer cooking time and less flavor. Instead, fill your slow cooker about two-thirds full.

Cook on low as often as you can. Using your slow cooker on high heat can result in stringy meat and dry, overcooked dishes with little flavor. Cooking on low or medium preserves the tenderness, moisture, and nutrients.

Essential Pantry Ingredients

In the recipes, you may notice that many ingredients are repeatedly used as staples. Consider keeping these ingredients on hand to make prep faster and easier.

Beans (black beans and white beans): Stock up on these fiber-rich legumes for delicious soups, stews, and vegetarian dishes.

Broths (homemade or store-bought): Broths serve as the base for many slow cooker recipes, so keeping chicken or vegetable broth on hand is essential at every stage of your recovery. Either make it yourself and freeze it or keep a store-bought version stocked in your pantry.

Brown rice: Rice is a staple in many slow cooker dishes due to its hearty taste and texture. Keep rice on hand for poultry dishes or as a quick and healthy side.

Dried herbs (cilantro, dill, oregano, parsley): You will likely be using an herb or herb mix in nearly all your slow cooker meals. Rather than scrambling to find them last minute at the grocery store, keep them on hand at all times.

Extra-virgin olive oil: Olive oil is an excellent cooking oil that adds depth and flavor to many slow cooker recipes.

Garlic: Because garlic is used so frequently, you may find it convenient to keep a jar of minced garlic on hand for quick and easy prep.

Potatoes: These mineral- and fiber-rich carbs are excellent for digestion when cooked to the proper texture in the soft-foods and general-foods stages.

Rolled oats: Keep these on hand for making breakfast and dessert recipes.

Spices (cinnamon, turmeric, cayenne, red pepper flakes, allspice, chili powder): Toward the end of your recovery, there will be some recipes that call for spices or spice mixes. Keep these on hand to make prep simple and fast.

Whole-grain pasta: Toward the end of your recovery, you may be making more recipes with pasta as your carbohydrate. Keeping a couple of varieties on hand provides for a fiber- and mineral-rich starch option.

Time-Saving Tips

Even though using a slow cooker is known to reduce prep time for meals, there are still even more ways to reduce prep time and make your use of the slow cooker as easy as possible. Making this process even easier will be particularly important during the earlier stages of your recovery.

Take advantage of batch-cooking. Any of the bean, vegetable, and basics recipes will be great to batch-cook on the weekends for easy weeknight meals.

Prep ingredients the night before. Chopping and prepping ingredients the night before is a great time-saver, so in the morning, all you need to do is combine the ingredients and press start.

Choose recipes that don't require precooking steps or intermediate steps. Any precooking steps or intermediate steps add to your total prep time. The most straightforward way to reduce prep time is to choose recipes that only require combining ingredients and turning the slow cooker on, like Apple Pie Overnight Oats (page 22), Breakfast Strawberry-Banana Quinoa (page 28), and Cajun Red Beans and Rice (page 38).

Lower the heat and cook for a longer period. Doing so will not only add depth and flavor to your dish but also allow you to go about your day (or night) without much interruption. Lowering the heat can mean going from 4 hours to 8 hours cooking time.

Choose recipes with fewer ingredients. This is a great way to reduce your grocery bill (and time spent at the store) and decrease the amount of time needed for prepping and cooking. Choose recipes with five to eight ingredients, such as Crustless Spinach and Feta Quiche (page 26), Slow Cooker Summer Vegetables (page 47), Creamy Homemade Greek Yogurt (page 90), and Cinnamon Apples and Pears (page 133).

Set, Forget, and Get Moving

Your habits and routines make the biggest difference in achieving and maintaining a healthy body weight and your overall health. Your slow cooker can help you create healthy, fast meals since it dramatically reduces prep time and your active cooking time. Another routine or habit that will help you achieve and maintain your weight goal is exercise. It doesn't have to be a marathon or even a 5K. Exercising regularly can include things that fit your fitness level:

Spend five minutes every hour performing warm-up movements. Starting simple and gentle is a great way to reduce the barrier to entry and get you moving. Commit to just five minutes at a time, and you may find yourself wanting to do more!

Take a 10-minute walk before and after work each day. Something simple and refreshing like a walk to start the day and end the day is a great stress buster, energizer, and metabolism booster. Aim to do this daily.

Find a physical activity you love (dancing, gardening, etc.), and commit to it a few times per week. Committing to something you love promotes enjoyment and sustainability! Exercise doesn't have to be something you dread. Find a new or familiar active hobby, and practice it regularly.

Find exercises you can do from your couch. This is a great way to bust resistance to exercise! It couldn't be easier to get started. Arm or ab exercises can easily be done while you're watching TV and don't have to involve expensive equipment.

About the Recipes

Over the course of your recovery, you'll become familiar with the recipes throughout this cookbook. Then you'll have a wealth of staples and go-to favorites that will help you maintain a healthy lifestyle beyond your recovery!

A few things to keep in mind as you get started:

Yields: All the recipes were tested in a 6-quart oval slow cooker, the most popular option for home cooks. If you are using a smaller or larger model, keep in mind when adjusting recipes that your slow cooker should always be about two-thirds full. Inadequate fill will lead to burning and overcooking, whereas overfilling will lead to extended cooking times. Additionally, make sure that your liquid-to-solid ratios are consistent. Keeping these two tips in mind, you may want to reduce a recipe by a third for a 4-quart slow cooker or increase the recipe by a third for an 8-quart slow cooker. This general amount would not apply to any baking done in your slow cooker, however, due to the need for any baked good to set appropriately during cooking. Instead, it's recommended you use two slow cookers to double a baked good recipe.

Stage: Each recipe includes icons that indicate the stage(s) that the recipe is appropriate for. This will help provide clarity for you at each stage. These icons will also be included in the at-a-glance recipe table of contents. The four icons used in the book are:

 LIQUIDS   SOFT FOODS

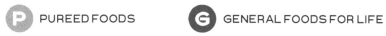 PUREED FOODS   GENERAL FOODS FOR LIFE

Serving Sizes: Each recipe includes specific serving sizes for each applicable stage.

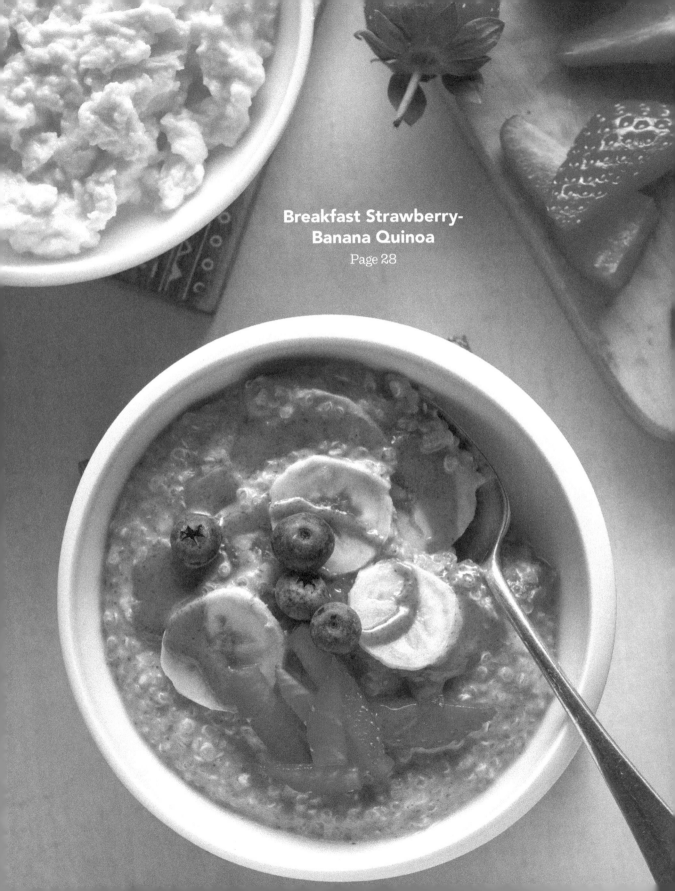

**Breakfast Strawberry-
Banana Quinoa**

Page 28

2

Breakfast & Beverages

L LIQUIDS   **S** SOFT FOODS   **P** PUREED FOODS   **G** GENERAL FOODS FOR LIFE

P **S** **G**

Apple Pie Overnight Oats

Prep time: 15 minutes
Cook time: 6 to 8 hours on low
SERVES 4

Enjoy the warm and sweet flavors of apple pie but with more soluble fiber and no added sugar. The soluble fiber from the oats will fill you up while providing a warm, soft, and gentle meal for your healing stomach.

1 to 2 tablespoons butter or coconut oil

4 cups unsweetened flax milk or coconut milk

1 cup rolled oats

1 to 2 cups (depending on how chunky you want it to be) chopped peeled apples or pears

2 tablespoons pure maple syrup

1 to 2 teaspoons ground cinnamon

1 teaspoon vanilla extract

½ cup nut butter, for topping (optional)

1. Coat the bottom and sides of a 6-quart slow cooker with the butter.

2. Add the milk, oats, apples, maple syrup, cinnamon, and vanilla. Mix well. Cover and cook on low for 6 to 8 hours, until the oats and apples are soft and the oatmeal has thickened.

3. Turn off the slow cooker. Serve the oats in a bowl topped with 2 tablespoons of nut butter per serving (if using).

4. Refrigerate leftovers for up to 3 days, or freeze for up to 1 month.

TIP

To make this recipe for your puree recovery stage, simply use an immersion blender to puree the oatmeal after cooking.

SERVING RECOMMENDATIONS

Pureed Foods: ¼–½ cup
Soft Foods: ½ cup
General Foods: 1 cup

Per serving: Calories: 205; Protein: 4g; Fat: 9g; Carbohydrates: 28g; Fiber: 4g; Sugar: 9g; Sodium: 47mg

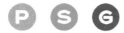

Veggie Lover's Breakfast Casserole

Prep time: 10 minutes
Cook time: 6 to 8 hours on low
SERVES 6 TO 8

Chock-full of colorful vegetables, this recipe is bursting with fiber, protein, iron, and B vitamins.

1 tablespoon extra-virgin olive oil

12 large eggs

¾ cup 2 percent milk

1 teaspoon sea salt

2 teaspoons Dijon mustard

¼ teaspoon ground black pepper

1 tablespoon onion powder

1 pound frozen hash browns

2 cups chopped or diced cored red, yellow, or orange bell peppers (or a combination)

1 (9.6-ounce) package cooked sausage, chopped into bite-size pieces

1½ cups shredded Cheddar cheese, divided

2 cups baby spinach

1. Coat the bottom of a 6-quart slow cooker with the olive oil.

2. In a large bowl, whisk together the eggs, milk, salt, mustard, black pepper, and onion powder.

3. Put the hash browns in the bottom of the slow cooker, followed, in order, by the bell peppers, sausage, 1 cup of cheese, the spinach, and the egg mixture. Do not stir. Cover and cook on low for 6 to 8 hours (do not exceed 8 hours), until the eggs have set.

4. Turn off the slow cooker. Remove the lid and add the remaining ½ cup of cheese. Replace the lid and let sit for about 5 minutes, until the cheese has melted. Serve warm.

5. Refrigerate leftovers for up to 5 days, or freeze for up to 1 month.

TIP

To make this recipe for your puree recovery stage, use an immersion blender to puree until smooth. For best results, puree single portions.

SERVING RECOMMENDATIONS

Pureed Foods: ¼–½ cup
Soft Foods: ½ cup
General Foods: 1 cup

Per serving: Calories: 484; Protein: 30g; Fat: 31g; Carbohydrates: 21g; Fiber: 3g; Sugar: 4g; Sodium: 868mg

Mixed Berry French Toast

Prep time: 15 minutes
Cook time: 4 hours on low
SERVES 6

This French toast recipe is great for brunch. You can prepare the ingredients in the slow cooker the night before, refrigerate them, then cook the French toast in the morning. On weekdays, simply cook it the night before and refrigerate it for the next morning.

Nonstick cooking spray, for coating the slow cooker

1 cup coconut sugar

4 tablespoons (½ stick) butter, melted

1¼ teaspoons ground cinnamon

12 whole-grain bread slices

1½ cups mixed fresh blueberries and raspberries, plus more for serving (optional)

6 large eggs

1½ cups 2 percent milk

1 tablespoon vanilla extract

½ teaspoon sea salt

¾ cup almond butter, for topping (optional)

¾ cup light whipped cream, for topping (optional)

1. Coat the bottom of a 6-quart slow cooker with cooking spray.

2. In a small bowl, mix together the sugar, butter, and cinnamon.

3. Spread one-third of the cinnamon-sugar butter on the bottom of the slow cooker.

4. Arrange 6 bread slices on top of the cinnamon-sugar butter.

5. Cover the bread with another third of the cinnamon-sugar butter, then sprinkle the berries over the top.

6. Layer the remaining 6 bread slices on top of the berries, and cover with the remaining third of the cinnamon-sugar butter.

7. In a medium bowl, whisk together the eggs, milk, vanilla, and salt.

8. Pour the egg mixture evenly over the bread layers. Do not stir. Cover and cook on low for 4 hours, until the French toast is golden brown and set on top.

9. Turn off the slow cooker. Serve the French toast with more berries (if using), 2 tablespoons of almond butter per serving (if using), or 2 tablespoons of light whipped cream per serving (if using) on top.

10. Refrigerate leftovers for up to 5 days, or freeze for up to 2 weeks.

MAKE IT A MEAL

Top with 1 tablespoon of peanut or almond butter, and serve with a scrambled egg on the side for added protein.

SERVING RECOMMENDATIONS

General Foods: 2 slices

Per serving: Calories: 593; Protein: 22g; Fat: 18g; Carbohydrates: 85g; Fiber: 10g; Sugar: 45g; Sodium: 640mg

P S G

Crustless Spinach and Feta Quiche

Prep time: 15 minutes
Cook time: 5 to 6 hours on low
SERVES 6

Meet your protein, B vitamin, and iron needs with this easy quiche that is also gentle on your healing stomach and excellent for the soft-foods phase of recovery. The feta ups the flavor ante while also contributing creamy texture with the eggs and milk. This recipe is great on its own or paired with fresh fruit or rice.

1 tablespoon extra-virgin olive oil

12 large eggs

1 cup whole-grain biscuit mix or whole-grain pancake and waffle mix

1 cup 2 percent milk

2 cups baby spinach

1½ cups crumbled feta cheese, plus more for topping (optional)

1 teaspoon garlic powder

½ teaspoon sea salt

1. Coat the bottom of a 6-quart slow cooker with the olive oil.

2. Add the eggs, biscuit mix, and milk. Whisk together until smooth.

3. Add the spinach, cheese, garlic powder, and salt. Mix well. Cover and cook on low for 5 to 6 hours, until the center of the quiche has set and the edges are golden brown.

4. Turn off the slow cooker. Serve the quiche with additional cheese on top, if desired. Do not top with cheese if you are in the pureed-foods stage.

5. Refrigerate any leftovers for up to 5 days, or freeze for up to 1 month.

TIP

To make this recipe for your puree recovery stage, use an immersion blender to puree until smooth. For best results, puree in single portions.

SERVING RECOMMENDATIONS

Pureed Foods: ¼–½ cup

Soft Foods: ½ cup

General Foods: 1 cup

Per serving: Calories: 367; Protein: 23g; Fat: 21g; Carbohydrates: 22g; Fiber: 0g; Sugar: 4g; Sodium: 941mg

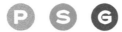

Vanilla-Maple Farina

Prep time: 5 minutes
Cook time: 8 hours on low
SERVES 4

This simple and sweet farina recipe is perfect for your pureed-foods recovery phase. It is both easy on your healing stomach and rich in calcium and iron. The milk increases protein and calcium content as well. Serve warm for any meal!

¾ cup Cream of Wheat

½ teaspoon sea salt

2 cups water

2 cups 2 percent milk

¾ teaspoon vanilla extract

¼ cup pure maple syrup, plus more for topping

1. In a 6-quart slow cooker, combine the Cream of Wheat, salt, water, milk, vanilla, and maple syrup. Cover and cook on low for 8 hours, until thick and creamy.

2. Turn off the slow cooker. Serve the farina warm, topped with maple syrup.

3. Refrigerate leftovers for up to 5 days, or freeze for up to 2 months.

TIP

When reheating, add 1 to 2 tablespoons of milk to reduce the thickness (this will thicken in the refrigerator).

SERVING RECOMMENDATIONS

Pureed Foods: ¼–½ cup
Soft Foods: ½ cup
General Foods: 1 cup

Per serving: Calories: 235; Protein: 7g; Fat: 3g; Carbohydrates: 44g; Fiber: 1g; Sugar: 18g; Sodium: 207mg

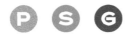

Breakfast Strawberry-Banana Quinoa

Prep time: 10 minutes
Cook time: 6 to 8 hours on low
SERVES 6

Fresh strawberries and bananas meet in this hot cereal breakfast to make for a comforting, easy, and filling meal. Quinoa provides essential minerals, protein, and fiber, while the nut butter and plant-based milk offer healthy fats to keep you full until lunch. This is great for the soft-foods phase of recovery.

1½ cups quinoa, rinsed

3 cups unsweetened cashew, coconut, or flax milk

2 cups fresh strawberries, halved, plus for more topping (optional)

1 large banana, peeled and sliced, plus more for topping (optional)

3 tablespoons almond butter or peanut butter

1. In a 6-quart slow cooker, mix together the quinoa, milk, strawberries, banana, and nut butter. Cover and cook on low for 6 to 8 hours, until the liquid has been absorbed.

2. Turn off the slow cooker. Serve the quinoa warm, topped with additional berries or banana (if using).

3. Refrigerate leftovers for up to 1 week, or freeze for up to 1 month.

MAKE IT A MEAL

Serve with an additional 2 tablespoons of nut or seed butter or with 2 scrambled eggs to add protein.

TIP

Choose blueberries or raspberries in place of the strawberries and a peach instead of the banana. This dish is also great with a little honey drizzled over the top.

SERVING RECOMMENDATIONS

Pureed Foods: ¼–½ cup

Soft Foods: ½ cup

General Foods: 1 cup

Per serving: Calories: 282; Protein: 8g; Fat: 11g; Carbohydrates: 38g; Fiber: 5g; Sugar: 6g; Sodium: 48mg

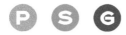

Bean Stew with Turkey Bacon and Potatoes

Prep time: 10 minutes
Cook time: 8 hours on low
SERVES 8

This savory and smooth stew is protein- and fiber-rich to support your nutritional needs during the final phase of your recovery. The flavor continues to develop after cooking, so the leftovers are delicious. Serve warm with a slice of whole-grain bread for a comforting, calming meal any time of day.

1 teaspoon onion powder

2 teaspoons minced garlic

1 (12-ounce) package turkey bacon, chopped

2 cups canned diced and peeled white potatoes, drained

3 cups dried white and kidney beans, rinsed

1 teaspoon sea salt

½ teaspoon ground black pepper

8 cups Savory Chicken Broth (page 144) or store-bought chicken broth

1. In a 6-quart slow cooker, mix together the onion powder, garlic, bacon, potatoes, beans, salt, black pepper, and broth. Cook on low for 8 hours.

2. Turn off the slow cooker. Serve the stew warm.

3. Refrigerate leftovers for up to 5 days, or freeze for up to 1 month.

TIP

To make this recipe for your puree recovery stage, let the soup cool until slightly warm or room temperature, then transfer one serving at a time to a blender or food processor and puree until smooth.

SERVING RECOMMENDATIONS

Pureed Foods: ¼–½ cup
Soft Foods: ½ cup
General Foods: 1 cup

Per serving: Calories: 392; Protein: 27g; Fat: 8g; Carbohydrates: 54g; Fiber: 13g; Sugar: 3g; Sodium: 715mg

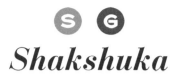

Shakshuka

Prep time: 15 minutes
Cook time: 7 hours on low and 25 minutes on high
SERVES 6 TO 8

I've reduced the spice level in this recipe to create a recovery-friendly yet flavorful savory breakfast. Rich in protein, B vitamins, antioxidants, and fiber, this recipe is the full package. Serve it for breakfast, lunch, or dinner to meet your protein and vegetable needs.

3 tablespoons extra-virgin olive oil

1 medium yellow or white onion, chopped

2 cups chopped and cored red and orange bell peppers, preferably 1 cup each

1 tablespoon minced garlic

1 (28-ounce) container plus 1 (15-ounce) container crushed tomatoes

½ teaspoon sea salt

½ teaspoon ground black pepper

1 teaspoon paprika

1 teaspoon dried oregano

1 teaspoon ground cumin

8 large eggs

1½ to 2 cups feta cheese, for topping (optional)

1½ to 2 cups pitted olives, for topping (optional)

6 to 8 teaspoons chopped fresh parsley, for topping (optional)

1. In a 6-quart slow cooker, mix together the olive oil, onion, bell peppers, garlic, tomatoes, salt, black pepper, paprika, oregano, and cumin. Cover and cook on low for 7 hours, until the mixture has thickened slightly (the sauce may also be bubbly).

2. Increase the heat to high. Remove the lid and, using a ¼-cup measuring cup, make 8 indentations in the top of the mixture. Fill each indentation with 1 egg. Replace the lid and cook for 20 to 25 minutes, until the egg whites have set.

3. Turn off the slow cooker. Serve the shakshuka warm, topped with any combination of ¼ cup of cheese per serving (if using), ¼ cup of olives per serving (if using), or 1 teaspoon of chopped parsley per serving (if using).

4. Refrigerate leftovers for up to 3 days, or freeze for up to 2 weeks.

SERVING RECOMMENDATIONS

Soft Foods: ½ cup
General Foods: 1 cup

Per serving: Calories: 228; Protein: 12g; Fat: 14g; Carbohydrates: 16g; Fiber: 4g; Sugar: 9g; Sodium: 458mg

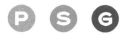

Breakfast Protein Soup

Prep time: 15 minutes
Cook time: 5 to 6 hours on low or 4 hours on high
SERVES 6 TO 8

This recipe combines all the best flavors of a savory breakfast and the comforting texture of a hot soup. Rich in protein, B vitamins, and iron, this meal safely provides all your most essential nutritional needs for your soft-foods stage of healing.

1 tablespoon extra-virgin olive oil

5 cups chopped cooked sausage

1 (12-ounce) package turkey bacon, chopped

2½ cups canned diced and peeled white potatoes, drained

1 (15-ounce) can diced tomatoes, drained

4 cups Savory Chicken Broth (page 144) or store-bought chicken broth

2 teaspoons minced garlic

1 (1-ounce) packet Hollandaise sauce mix

6 to 16 scrambled eggs or egg whites (optional)

1. In a 6-quart slow cooker, mix together the olive oil, sausage, bacon, potatoes, and tomatoes.

2. In a medium bowl, combine the broth, garlic, and Hollandaise sauce mix. Mix well.

3. Pour the broth mixture into the slow cooker and stir. Cover and cook on low for 5 to 6 hours or on high for 4 hours.

4. Turn off the slow cooker. Serve the soup warm, topped with 1 or 2 scrambled eggs or egg whites per serving (if using).

5. Refrigerate any leftovers for up to 1 week, or freeze for up to 1 month.

TIP

For your puree recovery stage, let the soup cool until slightly warm or room temperature, then transfer one serving at a time to a blender or food processor and puree until smooth.

SERVING RECOMMENDATIONS

Pureed Foods: ¼–½ cup
Soft Foods: ½ cup

General Foods: 1 cup

Per serving: Calories: 420; Protein: 22g; Fat: 28g; Carbohydrates: 20g; Fiber: 3g; Sugar: 3g; Sodium: 1,322mg

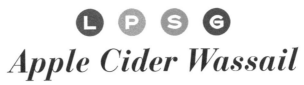

Apple Cider Wassail

Prep time: 10 minutes
Cook time: 6 to 8 hours on low
SERVES 8 TO 10

This comforting wassail is perfect for the liquids stage of your healing and recovery. The no-sugar-added juices will also help support your weight-management goals. Although best warm, this wassail is also delicious served cold. It will also reheat well on your stove over low heat.

8 cups apple cider

2 cups no-sugar-added orange juice

1 cup no-sugar-added cranberry juice

5 cinnamon sticks

10 whole cloves

½ teaspoon ground nutmeg

½ teaspoon ground ginger

1 orange, sliced

1 apple, sliced

¼ cup cranberries

1. In a 6-quart slow cooker, mix together the apple cider, orange juice, cranberry juice, cinnamon sticks, cloves, nutmeg, and ginger. Cover and cook on low for 6 to 8 hours, until the mixture is heated through and fragrant.

2. When there are 20 to 30 minutes left of cooking time, remove the lid and add the orange, apple, and cranberries. Replace the lid and continue cooking for the remaining 20 to 30 minutes.

3. Turn off the slow cooker. Serve the wassail warm in mugs. If you are in the liquids stage, strain and discard the solids before serving.

4. Refrigerate leftovers for up to 1 week, or freeze for up to 1 month.

SERVING RECOMMENDATIONS

Liquids: ¼–½ cup
Pureed Foods: ¼–½ cup
Soft Foods: ½ cup
General Foods: 1 cup

Per serving: Calories: 174; Protein: 1g; Fat: 1g; Carbohydrates: 42g; Fiber: 1g; Sugar: 36g; Sodium: 12mg

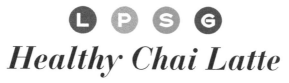

Healthy Chai Latte

Prep time: 10 minutes
Cook time: 4 hours on low
SERVES 8

This warm latte surprisingly contains 7 to 8 grams of protein per cup (from the milk!), and it's a great way to consume your required liquids early on in recovery while also supporting your protein needs. This recipe also reheats well on the stove over low heat.

8 chai tea bags

2 or 3 decaf black tea bags

8 cups 2 percent milk

3 tablespoons pure maple syrup or liquid stevia

Ground cinnamon, for topping (optional)

1 cup light whipped cream, for topping (optional)

1. Put the chai tea bags and black tea bags in a 6-quart slow cooker, then pour in the milk and maple syrup and stir. Cover and cook on low for 4 hours, until heated through and fragrant.

2. Turn off the slow cooker. Discard the tea bags. Serve the latte warm in mugs, topped with a sprinkle of ground cinnamon (if using) or 2 tablespoons of light whipped cream per serving (if using). Do not use the toppings if you are in the liquids stage.

3. Refrigerate leftovers for up to 1 week, or freeze for up to 1 month.

TIP

If you are sensitive to caffeine, use decaf black tea bags.

SERVING RECOMMENDATIONS

Liquids: ¼–½ cup
Pureed Foods: ¼–½ cup
Soft Foods: ½ cup
General Foods: 1 cup

Per serving: Calories: 142; Protein: 8g; Fat: 5g; Carbohydrates: 17g; Fiber: 0g; Sugar: 17g; Sodium: 116mg

L P S G

Warm Cran-Pineapple Punch

Prep time: 10 minutes
Cook time: 4 hours on low
SERVES 8

This punch, perfect for the liquids stage, is easy and satisfying. If you need something in fewer than 4 hours, you can heat this, albeit with slightly less flavor, in about 2 hours. This punch also reheats well on the stove in about 10 minutes over low heat.

5 decaf black tea bags

1 cup no-sugar-added orange juice

1 cup no-sugar-added apple juice

2 cups chopped pineapple

5 cups apple cider

1 cup fresh cranberries

Ground cinnamon, for topping (optional)

1. In a 6-quart slow cooker, combine the tea bags, orange juice, apple juice, pineapple, apple cider, and cranberries. Mix well. Cover and cook on low for 4 hours, until the mixture is warm but not boiling.

2. Turn off the slow cooker. Discard the tea bags. Serve the punch warm in mugs with a sprinkle of cinnamon on top (if using). If you are in the liquids stage, strain and discard the solids before serving. Refrigerate leftovers for up to 1 week, or freeze for up to 1 month.

TIP

You can mix up the fruit and fruit juice ratios here, depending on the flavor you want. For example, if you don't want orange flavor, eliminate the orange juice and double the apple juice (or vice versa).

SERVING RECOMMENDATIONS

Liquids: ¼–½ cup
Pureed Foods: ¼–½ cup
Soft Foods: ½ cup
General Foods: 1 cup

Per serving: Calories: 190; Protein: 1g; Fat: 0g; Carbohydrates: 47g; Fiber: 2g; Sugar: 40g; Sodium: 11mg

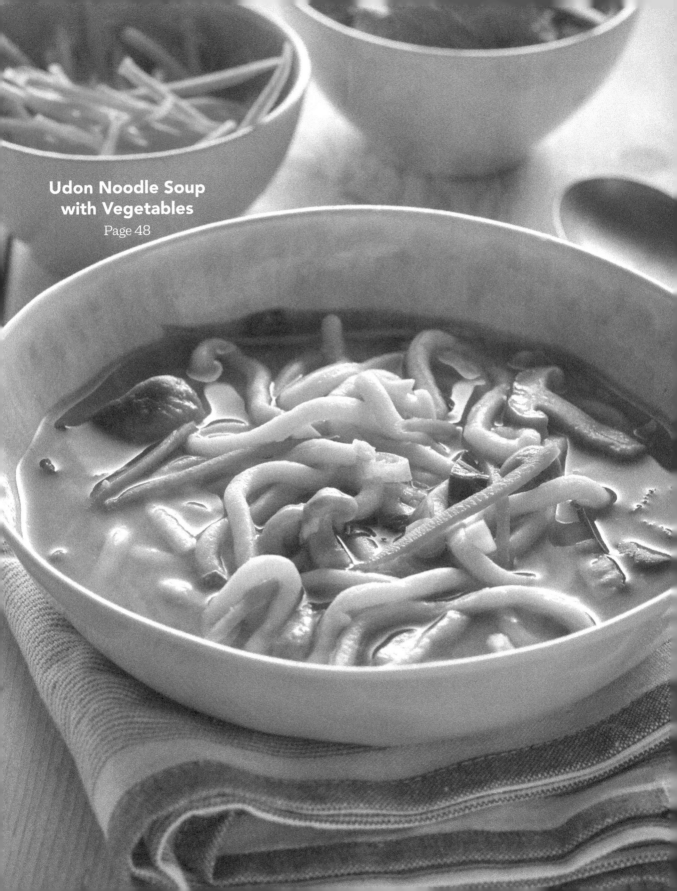

**Udon Noodle Soup
with Vegetables**

Page 48

3

Beans & Vegetables

Ⓛ LIQUIDS   SOFT FOODS   PUREED FOODS   GENERAL FOODS FOR LIFE

Cajun Red Beans and Rice

Prep time: 15 minutes
Cook time: 8 hours on low
SERVES 6 TO 8

With roots in Louisiana Creole cuisine, this spicy dish is easy and filling. Typically made on Mondays with leftovers from Sunday dinner, this recipe provides fiber to keep you full, complex carbohydrates for energy, protein to help your recovery, and antioxidants to support your overall health. It's perfect for the soft-foods stage of your recovery.

1 (14- to 16-ounce) can red kidney beans, drained and rinsed

4 cups Savory Chicken Broth (page 144) or store-bought chicken broth

6 cups water

1 pound andouille, chorizo, smoked beef sausage, or ham, sliced

1 medium yellow onion, chopped

1 orange or yellow bell pepper, cored and chopped

1 cup chopped celery

¼ cup minced garlic

1 teaspoon ground black pepper

2 tablespoons Creole seasoning

6 to 8 cups cooked brown or wild rice

1. Put the beans in the bottom of a 6-quart slow cooker, then pour the broth and water over the beans.

2. Add the sausage, onion, bell pepper, celery, garlic, black pepper, and Creole seasoning. Mix well. Cover and cook on low for 8 hours, until the beans are soft and easily mashed.

3. Turn off the slow cooker. Serve the beans warm over the rice.

4. Refrigerate leftovers for up to 1 week, or freeze for up to 1 month.

MAKE IT A MEAL

Serve with ¼ cup of grilled chicken breast or ¼ cup of more sausage on the side.

SERVING RECOMMENDATIONS

Soft Foods: ½ cup
General Foods: 1 cup

Per serving: Calories: 524; Protein: 19g; Fat: 27g; Carbohydrates: 53g; Fiber: 6g; Sugar: 4g; Sodium: 1,232mg

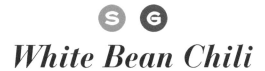

White Bean Chili

Prep time: 15 minutes
Cook time: 3 minutes on high and 6 to 8 hours on low
SERVES 8

My favorite things about this chili? It's easy and flavorful! It's full of protein and fiber from the beans, onion, and spinach. This chili is also particularly gentle on your healing stomach with its smooth texture, and the lack of tomatoes may be of benefit to you if you're struggling with acidity postsurgery.

2 tablespoons extra-virgin olive oil

¼ cup minced garlic

½ teaspoon onion powder

½ teaspoon garlic powder

1 tablespoon ground cumin

1 teaspoon chili powder

½ teaspoon paprika

1 medium yellow onion, chopped

2 (15-ounce) cans great northern beans, drained and rinsed

3 cups Savory Vegetable Broth (page 146) or store-bought vegetable broth

1 (10-ounce) package frozen chopped spinach

Sea salt

Ground black pepper

1 cup shredded mild Cheddar cheese, for topping (optional)

1 cup sour cream, for topping (optional)

Fresh cilantro, for topping (optional)

Freshly squeezed lime juice, for topping (optional)

1. In a 6-quart slow cooker, combine the olive oil, garlic, onion powder, garlic powder, cumin, chili powder, and paprika. Cook on high, stirring occasionally, for 2 to 3 minutes, until fragrant.

2. Add the onion and beans, then pour the broth over everything. Mix well.

3. Gently layer the spinach over the top. Do not mix; let the spinach stay on top to steam. Cover, reduce the heat to low, and cook for 6 to 8 hours (start checking for doneness after 6 hours), until the beans are soft and easily mashed.

4. Turn off the slow cooker. Season with salt and black pepper. Stir the spinach into the chili.

5. Top with any combination of 2 tablespoons of cheese per serving (if using); 2 tablespoons of sour cream per serving (if using); chopped cilantro (if using); or lime juice (if using). Serve warm.

CONTINUED →

6. Refrigerate leftovers for up to 5 days, or freeze for up to 2 months.

MAKE IT A MEAL

Serve with ¼ cup of chopped grilled chicken breast or chopped cooked ham toward the end of cooking time for additional protein.

SERVING RECOMMENDATIONS

Soft Foods: ½ cup
General Foods: 1 cup

Per serving: Calories: 136; Protein: 7g; Fat: 4g; Carbohydrates: 19g; Fiber: 6g; Sugar: 1g; Sodium: 79mg

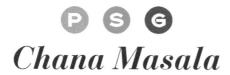

Chana Masala

Prep time: 10 minutes
Cook time: 3 minutes on high and 6 to 7 hours on low
SERVES 4 TO 6

Originating in northern India, this warming and satisfying dish is rich in flavor while still being gentle on your healing stomach. "Chana" means "chickpea," and "masala" refers to the array of spices used to create such rich flavor.

1 tablespoon extra-virgin olive oil

¼ cup garlic, minced

1 tablespoon grated fresh ginger

½ teaspoon sea salt

¼ teaspoon ground black pepper

2 tablespoons garam masala

½ teaspoon ground turmeric

1 medium onion, chopped

1 (28-ounce) can crushed tomatoes, drained

2 (15-ounce) cans chickpeas, drained and rinsed

2 cups Savory Vegetable Broth (page 146) or store-bought vegetable broth

1 to 1½ cups cooked basmati, brown, or wild rice

Chopped fresh cilantro, for topping (optional)

1. In a 6-quart slow cooker, combine the olive oil, garlic, ginger, salt, black pepper, garam masala, and turmeric. Cook on high, stirring occasionally, for 2 to 3 minutes, until fragrant.

2. Add the onion, tomatoes, and chickpeas, then pour the broth over everything. Mix well. Cover, reduce the heat to low, and cook for 6 to 7 hours (start checking for doneness after 6 hours), until the chickpeas are soft and easily mashed.

3. Turn off the slow cooker. Serve the chana masala with the rice, topped with cilantro (if using). Refrigerate leftovers for up to 5 days, or freeze for up to 2 months.

TIP

To make this recipe for your puree recovery stage, use an immersion blender to puree until smooth. For best results, puree in single portions.

SERVING RECOMMENDATIONS

Pureed Foods: ¼–½ cup

Soft Foods: ½ cup

General Foods: 1 cup

Per serving: Calories: 344; Protein: 15g; Fat: 8g; Carbohydrates: 58g; Fiber: 15g; Sugar: 12g; Sodium: 386mg

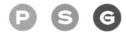

Chili-Cumin Pinto Beans

Prep time: 15 minutes
Cook time: 6 to 7 hours on low
SERVES 8 TO 10

This dish may be one of the most versatile of the bean dishes. Its savory and mildly spicy flavor means it pairs well with not only rice but also potatoes, chili, burritos, and tacos. Its soft texture is also comforting and gentle on your healing stomach. Serving with pico de gallo is a must for the most dynamic flavor!

2 (16-ounce) cans pinto beans, drained and rinsed

2 tablespoons extra-virgin olive oil

1 medium yellow onion, chopped

4 cups Savory Chicken Broth (page 144) or store-bought chicken broth

3 tablespoons minced garlic

2 teaspoons ground cumin

1 tablespoon chili powder

Sea salt

Ground black pepper

2 to 2½ cups cooked white rice

Sliced avocado, for topping (optional)

Chopped fresh cilantro, for topping (optional)

1 to 1¼ cups crumbled queso fresco, for topping (optional)

1 to 1¼ cups shredded Monterey Jack cheese, for topping (optional)

1 to 1¼ cups tablespoons pico de gallo, for topping (optional)

1. In a 6-quart slow cooker, combine the beans, olive oil, onion, broth, garlic, cumin, and chili powder. Mix well. Cover and cook on low for 6 to 7 hours (start checking for doneness after 6 hours), until the beans are soft and easily mashed.

2. Turn off the slow cooker. Season with salt and black pepper. Stir. Serve the beans over ¼ cup of rice per serving and with your choice of sliced avocado (if using), chopped cilantro (if using), 2 tablespoons of queso fresco per serving (if using), 2 tablespoons of Monterey Jack cheese per serving (if using), or 2 tablespoons of pico de gallo per serving (if using). Do not use the toppings if you are in the pureed-foods stage.

3. Refrigerate leftovers for up to 5 days, or freeze for up to 2 months.

Serve with shredded cheese and shredded chicken over rice or on top of chili.

TIP

You can easily turn these into refried beans by mashing the beans using a potato masher, or you can puree them for a smoother texture if you want to enjoy these at the puree stage.

SERVING RECOMMENDATIONS

Pureed Foods: ¼–½ cup
Soft Foods: ½ cup
General Foods: 1 cup

Per serving: Calories: 188; Protein: 7g; Fat: 4g; Carbohydrates: 31g; Fiber: 7g; Sugar: 1g; Sodium: 71mg

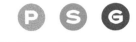

Easy Mashed Potatoes

Prep time: 10 minutes
Cook time: 2 to 3 hours on low
SERVES 8 TO 10

Mashed potatoes have never been so easy! This simple recipe is perfect for your pureed-foods stage (as well as your soft- and general-foods phases). The cottage cheese and yogurt add essential protein, calcium, and B vitamins for nutritional balance and enrichment.

Nonstick cooking spray, for coating the slow cooker

1¾ cups 2 percent milk

3½ cups water, heated in the microwave until hot to the touch

8 ounces cream cheese, cubed

8 tablespoons (1 stick) butter, at room temperature

½ cup 2 percent cottage cheese

¼ cup 2 percent plain yogurt

4 cups potato flakes (instant mashed potatoes)

1 teaspoon sea salt

1. Coat the bottom and sides of a 6-quart slow cooker with cooking spray.

2. Add the milk, water, cream cheese, butter, cottage cheese, and yogurt. Whisk until smooth. Stir in the potato flakes and salt. Cover and cook on low for 2 to 3 hours, until heated through.

3. Turn off the slow cooker. Serve the potatoes warm as a side dish with your favorite protein.

4. Refrigerate leftovers for up to 5 days, or freeze for up to 2 months.

TIP

In your pureed-foods phase, serve with ¼ cup of cottage cheese or yogurt on the side for more protein.

SERVING RECOMMENDATIONS

Pureed Foods: ¼–½ cup
Soft Foods: ½ cup
General Foods: 1 cup

Per serving: Calories: 333; Protein: 7g; Fat: 23g; Carbohydrates: 24g; Fiber: 1g; Sugar: 4g; Sodium: 344mg

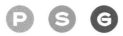

Savory Mashed Root Vegetables

Prep time: 15 minutes
Cook time: 3 minutes on high and 6 to 7 hours on low
SERVES 6 TO 8

Boost your vegetable, fiber, and antioxidant intake with this warm, savory dish. It combines well with almost any roasted, baked, or grilled protein, and its soft texture makes it particularly great for your soft-foods recovery stage.

1 tablespoon butter

1 tablespoon extra-virgin olive oil

2 tablespoons minced garlic

1 teaspoon sea salt

½ teaspoon ground black pepper

1½ teaspoons dried thyme

2 pounds mixed root vegetables (any combination of sweet potatoes, white potatoes, carrots, turnips, and parsnips), peeled and chopped

¼ cup Savory Vegetable Broth (page 146) or store-bought vegetable broth

⅓ cup 2 percent milk, whole milk, or half-and-half

Sliced scallions, for topping (optional)

¾ to 1 cup sour cream, for topping (optional)

1. In a 6-quart slow cooker, combine the butter, olive oil, garlic, salt, black pepper, and thyme. Cook on high, stirring frequently, for 2 to 3 minutes, until fragrant.

2. Add the root vegetables, broth, and milk. Mix well. Cover and cook on low for 6 to 7 hours (start checking for doneness after 6 hours), until the root vegetables are easily mashed.

3. Turn off the slow cooker. Either transfer the contents to a large mixing bowl and mash coarsely using a hand masher, or transfer to a blender and puree.

4. Serve the vegetables warm, topped with scallions (if using) and 2 tablespoons of sour cream per serving (if using). Do not use the scallions if you are at the pureed-foods stage.

5. Refrigerate leftovers for up to 5 days, or freeze for up to 1 month.

MAKE IT A MEAL

Serve with 2 ounces of rotisserie-style chicken or fish.

CONTINUED →

Savory Mashed Root Vegetables CONTINUED

TIP

If in the general-foods stage, you can skip the mashing process, and serve as is.

SERVING RECOMMENDATIONS

Pureed Foods: ¼–½ cup
Soft Foods: ½ cup
General Foods: 1 cup

Per serving: Calories: 179; Protein: 3g; Fat: 5g; Carbohydrates: 32g; Fiber: 5g; Sugar: 7g; Sodium: 299mg

Slow Cooker Summer Vegetables

Prep time: 15 minutes
Cook time: 3 minutes on high and 4 to 5 hours on low
SERVES 6 TO 8

This super easy dish is flexible on cooking time while still delivering on flavor. Fiber and anti-oxidants abound with the variety of vegetables, and their soft texture makes them perfect for your soft-foods recovery stage. You can try different vegetable combinations each time to mix up flavor and texture as desired.

½ cup extra-virgin olive oil

½ cup balsamic vinegar

2 tablespoons chopped fresh basil leaves

1 tablespoon dried thyme

1 (16-ounce) can chopped or diced tomatoes, drained

1 cup chopped white onion

2½ cups sliced or chopped cored orange and yellow bell peppers

3 cups sliced peeled zucchini

1. In a 6-quart slow cooker, combine the olive oil, vinegar, basil, and thyme. Cook on high, stirring frequently, for 2 to 3 minutes, until fragrant.

2. Add the tomatoes, onion, bell peppers, and zucchini. Mix well. Cover, reduce the heat to low, and cook for 4 to 5 hours, until the vegetables are soft.

3. Turn off the slow cooker. Serve the vegetables warm on their own or as a side dish.

4. Refrigerate leftovers for up to 3 days, or freeze for up to 1 month.

MAKE IT A MEAL

Serve with 2 ounces of rotisserie-style chicken or fish and rice.

SERVING RECOMMENDATIONS

Soft Foods: ½ cup
General Foods: ½–1 cup

Per serving: Calories: 223; Protein: 2g; Fat: 19g; Carbohydrates: 13g; Fiber: 3g; Sugar: 9g; Sodium: 99mg

Udon Noodle Soup with Vegetables

Prep time: 15 minutes
Cook time: 3 minutes on high and 6 hours on low
SERVES 4

A popular staple of Japanese cuisine, udon is versatile and can be served hot or cold. It is theorized that udon originated in China in the 700s, but it did not become more popular until the 1600s. These noodles are compatible with a variety of other ingredients and dishes, making them an easy addition to many meals.

2 tablespoons extra-virgin olive oil

2 scallions, both white and green parts, chopped

1 tablespoon chopped peeled fresh ginger

2 tablespoons minced garlic

1 cup sliced shiitake mushrooms

2 tablespoons low-sodium soy sauce or coconut aminos

6 cups Savory Vegetable Broth (page 146) or store-bought vegetable broth

2 teaspoons red or white miso

1 cup chopped bok choy

8 to 10 ounces dried udon

Fresh spinach and shredded carrots, for topping (optional)

1. In a 6-quart slow cooker, combine the olive oil, scallions, ginger, garlic, mushrooms, and soy sauce. Cook on high, stirring frequently, for 2 to 3 minutes, until fragrant.

2. Pour in the broth and stir.

3. Add the miso and stir until dissolved.

4. Add the bok choy and udon. Mix thoroughly (make sure the udon is fully submerged). Cover, reduce the heat to low, and cook for 6 hours, until the udon is cooked.

5. Turn off the slow cooker. Serve the noodle soup warm over a handful of fresh spinach (if using) and a handful of shredded carrots (if using). Do not add the carrots if you are in the soft-foods stage.

6. Refrigerate leftovers for up to 1 week, or freeze for up to 2 months.

Serve with 2 ounces of rotisserie-style chicken or fish on the side.

TIP

Use rice noodles or soba noodles; tamari or coconut aminos; and a rice-, millet-, or buckwheat-based miso to make this gluten-free.

SERVING RECOMMENDATIONS

Soft Foods: ½ cup
General Foods: ½–1 cup

Per serving: Calories: 293; Protein: 9g; Fat: 8g; Carbohydrates: 48g; Fiber: 4g; Sugar: 2g; Sodium: 480mg

(S) (G)

Cheesy Cauliflower, Broccoli, and Carrots

Prep time: 10 minutes
Cook time: 4 to 5 hours on low
SERVES 8 TO 10

This vegetable side is a surprising protein powerhouse! Using Greek yogurt in place of cream boosts the protein content and provides essential B vitamins and calcium.

3 cups fresh broccoli florets

3 cups fresh cauliflower florets

2 cups baby carrots

1 (8-ounce) container plain 2 percent Greek yogurt

1½ cups shredded sharp Cheddar cheese, divided

1 cup shredded mozzarella cheese, shredded provolone cheese, or a mix of both

1 cup 2 percent milk

1 tablespoon minced garlic

1 tablespoon minced onion

Sea salt

Ground black pepper

1. In a 6-quart slow cooker, combine the broccoli, cauliflower, and carrots.

2. In a large bowl, whisk together the yogurt, ¾ cup of Cheddar cheese, the mozzarella cheese, milk, garlic, and onion.

3. Pour the yogurt mixture over the vegetables and mix well. Cover and cook on low for 4 to 5 hours, until the vegetables are soft.

4. Remove the lid and sprinkle the remaining ¾ cup of Cheddar cheese over the top. Replace the lid and cook for an additional 5 to 10 minutes, until the cheese has melted.

5. Turn off the slow cooker. Season with salt and black pepper. Serve the vegetables warm. Refrigerate leftovers for up to 5 days, or freeze for up to 1 month.

SERVING RECOMMENDATIONS

Soft Foods: ½ cup
General Foods: ½–1 cup

Per serving: Calories: 196; Protein: 13g; Fat: 12g; Carbohydrates: 11g; Fiber: 3g; Sugar: 6g; Sodium: 320mg

Savory Collard Greens

Prep time: 15 minutes
Cook time: 10 minutes on high and 7 hours on low
SERVES 8 TO 10

Collard greens, whose origins lie in the Mediterranean, have been popular in the American South for centuries. Rich in anti-inflammatory chlorophyll, fiber, and essential vitamins and minerals, these greens are a perfect side dish during your soft-foods stage.

3 tablespoons extra-virgin olive oil

8 bacon slices, chopped

1 cup chopped or diced cooked ham

3 cups Savory Chicken Broth (page 144) or store-bought chicken broth

1 tablespoon coconut sugar

2 tablespoons apple cider vinegar

¼ teaspoon red pepper flakes

8 cups (2 pounds) collard greens, ribs and stems removed, torn into bite-size pieces

Sea salt

Ground black pepper

1. Pour the olive oil into a 6-quart slow cooker, then add the bacon. Cook on high, stirring frequently, for 2 to 3 minutes, until the bacon is crackling.

2. Add the ham, broth, sugar, vinegar, and red pepper flakes. Stir and cook for an additional 2 to 3 minutes.

3. Add the collard greens 1 cup at a time, stirring and letting the pieces wilt with each addition. Cover, reduce the heat to low, and cook for 7 hours, until the collard greens are soft and cooked through.

4. Turn off the slow cooker. Season with salt and black pepper. Serve the greens warm using a slotted spoon to allow the extra liquid to drain.

5. Refrigerate leftovers for up to 5 days, or freeze for up to 2 months.

CONTINUED →

Savory Collard Greens CONTINUED

MAKE IT A MEAL

Serve with ¼ cup of Chili-Cumin Pinto Beans (page 42) and 2 ounces of rotisserie-style chicken or fish on the side.

TIP

Substitute kale, turnip, or mustard greens for the collard greens (in the same amount) if desired.

SERVING RECOMMENDATIONS

Soft Foods: ½ cup
General Foods: ½–1 cup

Per serving: Calories: 194; Protein: 8g; Fat: 17g; Carbohydrates: 4g; Fiber: 1g; Sugar: 2g; Sodium: 393mg

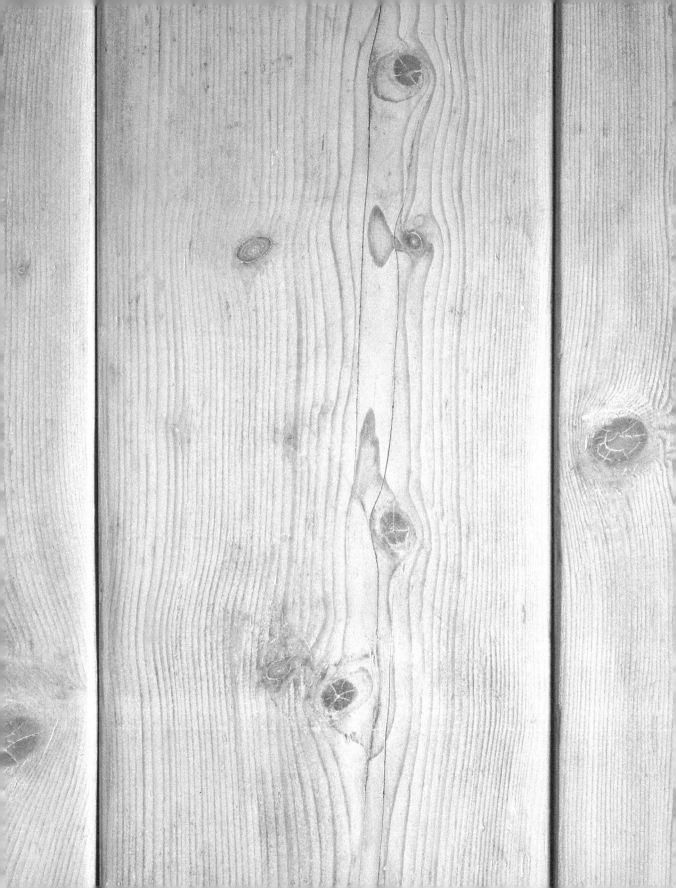

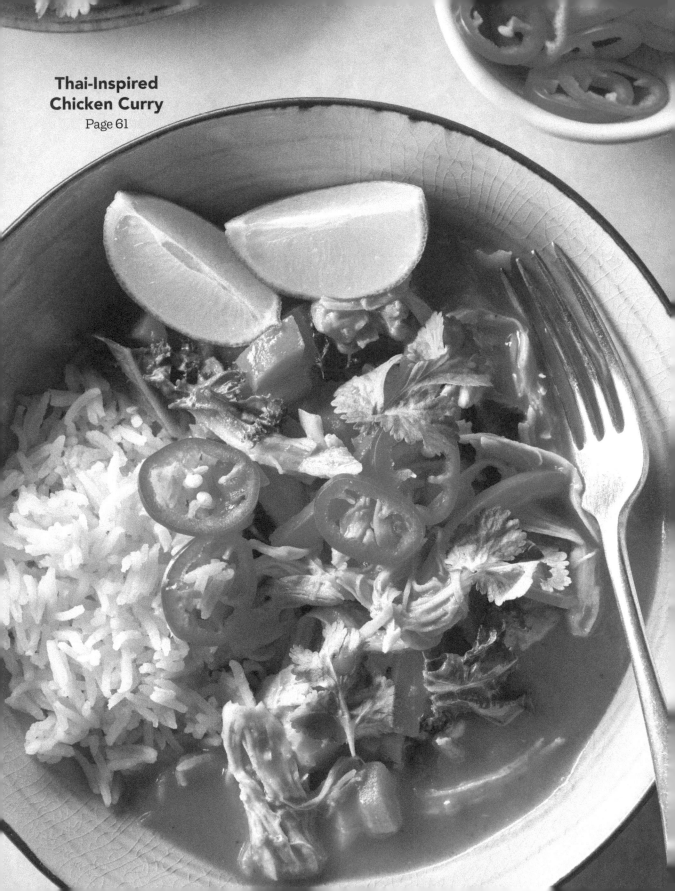

**Thai-Inspired
Chicken Curry**
Page 61

4

Soups, Stews & Chilis

L LIQUIDS **S** SOFT FOODS **P** PUREED FOODS **G** GENERAL FOODS FOR LIFE

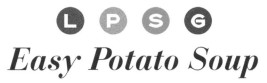

Easy Potato Soup

Prep time: 15 minutes
Cook time: 7½ to 8 hours on low
SERVES 10

Get your magnesium, calcium, and potassium needs met during your liquids stage with this creamy potato soup. If you want more texture or fullness during your soft- and general-foods stages, don't strain the solids after blending.

3 pounds fingerling potatoes, peeled and halved

2 teaspoons minced garlic

1 small white onion, chopped

1½ teaspoons sea salt

½ teaspoon ground black pepper

4 cups Savory Chicken Broth (page 144), Savory Vegetable Broth (page 146), or store-bought broth

2 cups 2 percent milk

1 cup shredded Cheddar cheese

1. In a 6-quart slow cooker, combine the potatoes, garlic, onion, salt, black pepper, and broth.

2. Cover and cook on low for 7 hours, until the potatoes are soft.

3. Remove the lid and stir in the milk and cheese. Replace the lid and cook for an additional 30 minutes to 1 hour, until the soup is heated through and the cheese has melted.

4. Turn off the slow cooker. Using an immersion blender, blend the soup until smooth. Pour through a strainer into a separate container, and discard any lumps or bits. Serve warm.

5. Refrigerate leftovers for up to 5 days, or freeze for up to 2 months.

SERVING RECOMMENDATIONS

Liquids: ¼–½ cup
Pureed Foods: ¼–½ cup
Soft Foods: ½ cup
General Foods: 1 cup

Per serving: Calories: 179; Protein: 7g; Fat: 5g; Carbohydrates: 27g; Fiber: 3g; Sugar: 4g; Sodium: 279mg

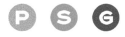

Comforting Beef Stew

Prep time: 15 minutes
Cook time: 4 minutes on high and 7½ to 8 hours on low
SERVES 8

A favorite comfort food, this beef stew will not disappoint. It is rich in protein, B vitamins, fiber, and flavor and is a meal in itself. Not to mention, the rich and savory aroma will fill your home.

2 tablespoons extra-virgin olive oil

2 pounds stew beef, cut into 1-inch cubes

Sea salt

Ground black pepper

1 pound fingerling potatoes, peeled and halved (3½ cups)

2 cups baby carrots

1 small onion, diced

3 tablespoons minced garlic

3 cups beef broth

1 (6-ounce) can tomato paste

1 teaspoon dried thyme

⅓ cup potato flakes

Chopped fresh parsley, for garnish (optional)

1. Coat the bottom of a 6-quart slow cooker with the olive oil.

2. Set the heat to high. Add the beef. Season with salt and black pepper. Sauté for 3 to 4 minutes, until browned.

3. Add the potatoes, carrots, onion, and garlic. Mix well. Stir in the broth, tomato paste, and thyme. Season with salt and black pepper. Mix well.

4. Cover, reduce the heat to low, and cook for 7 hours, until the vegetables are soft.

5. Remove the lid and stir in the potato flakes. Replace the lid and cook for an additional 30 minutes to 1 hour, until thickened.

6. Turn off the slow cooker. Serve the stew warm, garnished with parsley (if using).

7. Refrigerate leftovers for up to 1 week, or freeze for up to 2 months.

TIP

To make this recipe for your puree recovery stage, transfer one serving at a time to a blender or food processor and puree until smooth.

CONTINUED →

Comforting Beef Stew CONTINUED

SERVING RECOMMENDATIONS

Pureed Foods: ¼–½ cup
Soft Foods: ½ cup
General Foods: 1 cup

Per serving: Calories: 258; Protein: 28g; Fat: 8g; Carbohydrates: 20g; Fiber: 3g;
Sugar: 5g; Sodium: 151mg

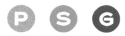

Tuscan Chicken and White Bean Stew

Prep time: 15 minutes
Cook time: 8 hours on low
SERVES 6 TO 8

As its name suggests, this robust stew—minus the chicken—originated in Tuscany, most likely in the Middle Ages. It was known originally as ribollita ("reboiled"), and the herbs, kale, and cannellini beans are essential components. The tender chicken and vegetables are perfect for your soft-foods recovery stage, and this stew reheats well on the stove.

1½ pounds boneless chicken thighs (about 6 whole thighs)

1 pound (3½ cups) halved peeled fingerling or baby potatoes

2 cups baby carrots

1 medium onion, diced

1 cup chopped celery

2 cups chopped kale

2 (15-ounce) cans white cannellini beans, drained and rinsed

1 (14½-ounce) can diced tomatoes, drained

2 tablespoons minced garlic

1 bay leaf

2 teaspoons dried oregano

2 teaspoons dried thyme

2 teaspoons dried rosemary

4 cups Savory Chicken Broth (page 144) or store-bought chicken broth

Sea salt

Ground black pepper

¾ to 1 cup grated Parmesan cheese, for topping (optional)

1. In a 6-quart slow cooker, combine the chicken, potatoes, carrots, onion, celery, kale, beans, tomatoes, garlic, bay leaf, oregano, thyme, rosemary, and broth. Mix well. Cover and cook on low for 8 hours, until the chicken has cooked through, the vegetables are soft, and the beans are easily mashed.

2. Remove the lid and remove the chicken. Shred using 2 forks. Return the meat to the slow cooker and stir. Season with salt and black pepper to taste.

3. Turn off the slow cooker. Discard the bay leaf. Serve the stew warm, topped with 2 tablespoons of cheese per serving (if using).

4. Refrigerate leftovers for up to 1 week, or freeze for up to 2 months.

CONTINUED →

Tuscan Chicken and White Bean Stew CONTINUED

CONTINUED

TIP

To make this recipe for your puree recovery stage, transfer one serving at a time to a blender or food processor and puree until smooth.

SERVING RECOMMENDATIONS

Pureed Foods: ¼–½ cup
Soft Foods: ½ cup
General Foods: 1 cup

Per serving: Calories: 480; Protein: 31g; Fat: 20g; Carbohydrates: 46g; Fiber: 11g; Sugar: 6g; Sodium: 253mg

Thai-Inspired Chicken Curry

Prep time: 15 minutes
Cook time: 7 hours on low
SERVES 6 TO 8

Thai curry is known for its aromatic qualities, largely from garlic, ginger, and onion. This dish also delivers on protein, antioxidants, and fiber from vegetables, and it is an excellent main dish for your soft-foods recovery stage.

3 cups Savory Chicken Broth (page 144) or store-bought chicken broth

5 tablespoons red Thai curry paste, such as Mae Ploy or Thai Kitchen

2⅔ cups canned coconut milk

1 tablespoon coconut sugar

1½ tablespoons low-sodium soy sauce or coconut aminos

1½ tablespoons minced fresh ginger

1 tablespoon fish sauce

¼ cup minced garlic

1½ pounds boneless, skinless chicken thighs, cut into bite-size pieces

1½ cups diced carrots

1 medium yellow onion, chopped

1 large red bell pepper, cored and sliced

2 cups chopped kale

1½ to 2 cups cooked basmati rice or cauliflower rice

Chopped fresh cilantro, freshly squeezed lime juice, or sliced chiles of your choice (such as Thai chiles or jalapeños), for topping (optional)

1. In a 6-quart slow cooker, combine the broth, curry paste, coconut milk, sugar, soy sauce, ginger, fish sauce, garlic, chicken, carrots, and onion. Cover and cook on low for 6 hours, until the chicken has cooked through and the vegetables are soft.

2. Remove the lid and add the bell pepper and kale. Replace the lid and cook for an additional 45 minutes to 1 hour.

3. Turn off the slow cooker. Serve the curry warm over the rice with cilantro, lime juice, or chiles (if using). Do not add the chiles if you are at the soft-foods stage.

4. Refrigerate leftovers for up to 5 days, or freeze for up to 1 month.

SERVING RECOMMENDATIONS

Soft Foods: ½ cup
General Foods: 1 cup

Per serving: Calories: 456; Protein: 28g; Fat: 27g; Carbohydrates: 28g; Fiber: 5g; Sugar: 6g; Sodium: 514mg

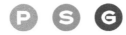

Pumpkin and Pork Stew

Prep time: 15 minutes
Cook time: 3 minutes on high and 5 hours 40 minutes on low
SERVES 6 TO 8

Smooth, savory, and slightly sweet, this richly flavored stew is perfect for cold days and during your soft-foods stage.

1 tablespoon extra-virgin olive oil

1 pound ground pork

1 large yellow onion, diced

1 (16-ounce) can pumpkin puree

2½ cups Savory Chicken Broth (page 144) or store-bought chicken broth

2 tablespoons minced garlic

½ teaspoon ground cinnamon

1 bay leaf

2 cups 2 percent milk

Sea salt

Ground black pepper

1. Coat the bottom of a 6-quart slow cooker with the olive oil.

2. Set the heat to high. Add the pork and cook, continuously stirring and breaking up the meat, for 2 to 3 minutes.

3. Add the onion, pumpkin, broth, garlic, cinnamon, and bay leaf. Mix well. Cover and cook on low for 5 hours, until the pork has cooked through.

4. Remove the lid and stir in the milk. Replace the lid and cook for an additional 30 to 40 minutes, until heated through.

5. Turn off the slow cooker. Season with salt and black pepper. Discard the bay leaf. Serve the stew warm. Refrigerate leftovers for up to 1 week, or freeze for up to 2 months.

TIP

To make this for your puree recovery stage, use a blender, food processor, or immersion blender to blend until smooth.

SERVING RECOMMENDATIONS

Pureed Foods: ¼–½ cup
Soft Foods: ½ cup

General Foods: 1 cup

Per serving: Calories: 300; Protein: 17g; Fat: 20g; Carbohydrates: 13g; Fiber: 3g; Sugar: 8g; Sodium: 138mg

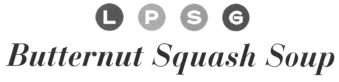

Butternut Squash Soup

Prep time: 15 minutes
Cook time: 5 to 6 hours on low
SERVES 6 TO 8

Nothing says fall quite like pumpkin and apples, especially together! The squash, carrots, onion, and apple will help you meet your vegetable and fiber goals. Add milk if you want to boost your protein and fat intake to feel full longer.

7 cups diced butternut squash

1 cup baby carrots

1 medium yellow onion, diced

1 Granny Smith apple, peeled, cored, and sliced

¼ cup minced garlic

½ teaspoon ground black pepper, plus more for seasoning

½ teaspoon ground cinnamon

½ teaspoon sea salt, plus more for seasoning

¼ teaspoon cayenne pepper

⅛ teaspoon ground nutmeg

4 cups Savory Vegetable Broth (page 146), Savory Chicken Broth (page 144), or store-bought broth

¼ cup 2 percent milk, coconut milk, or cashew cream (optional)

1. In a 6-quart slow cooker, combine the squash, carrots, onion, apple, garlic, black pepper, cinnamon, salt, cayenne, nutmeg, and broth. Cover and cook on low for 5 to 6 hours, until the squash is soft and easily mashed.

2. Turn off the slow cooker. Using an immersion blender, blend until smooth. Season with salt and pepper.

3. Stir in the milk (if using), and serve the soup warm. Refrigerate leftovers for up to 1 week, or freeze for up to 2 months.

SERVING RECOMMENDATIONS

Liquids: ¼ cup
Pureed Foods: ¼–½ cup
Soft Foods: ½ cup
General Foods: 1 cup

Per serving: Calories: 115; Protein: 3g; Fat: 0g; Carbohydrates: 29g; Fiber: 5g; Sugar: 8g; Sodium: 120mg

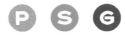

Spring Vegetable Minestrone

Prep time: 15 minutes
Cook time: 7 hours 20 minutes on low
SERVES 6 TO 8

Packed with vegetables, fiber, and flavor, this hearty classic is warm and satisfying. It's perfect for the soft-foods stage, but you can also bulk it up by adding ¼ cup more whole-grain pasta in step 2 for more fiber and minerals.

4 cups baby carrots

1 cup sliced celery

1 (28-ounce) can diced tomatoes, drained

1 medium yellow onion, diced

2 cups fresh green beans, cut into 2-inch pieces

2 (15-ounce) cans cannellini beans, drained and rinsed

3 tablespoons minced garlic

6 cups Savory Vegetable Broth (page 146) or store-bought broth

2 tablespoons Italian seasoning

½ teaspoon sea salt, plus more for seasoning

½ teaspoon ground black pepper, plus more for seasoning

1 cup whole-grain elbow pasta

¾ to 1 cup grated Parmesan cheese, for topping (optional)

1. In a 6-quart slow cooker, combine the carrots, celery, tomatoes, onion, green beans, cannellini beans, garlic, broth, Italian seasoning, salt, and black pepper. Mix well. Cover and cook on low for 7 hours, until the beans are easily mashed.

2. Remove the lid and stir in the pasta. Season with salt and pepper. Replace the lid and cook for an additional 15 to 20 minutes, until the pasta is tender.

3. Turn off the slow cooker. Top with 2 tablespoons of cheese per serving (if using), and serve the soup warm. Refrigerate leftovers for up to 1 week, or freeze for up to 2 months.

TIP

Blend until smooth with a blender, food processor, or immersion blender for your puree recovery stage.

SERVING RECOMMENDATIONS

Pureed Foods: ¼–½ cup
Soft Foods: ½ cup

General Foods: 1 cup

Per serving: Calories: 266; Protein: 13g; Fat: 1g; Carbohydrates: 54g; Fiber: 16g; Sugar: 10g; Sodium: 327mg

Hot and Sour Soup

Prep time: 15 minutes
Cook time: 7 hours on low and 30 minutes on high
SERVES 6 TO 8

This recipe is inspired by the dish originally from the Sichuan Province of China. Its standout characteristics are hot pepper and vinegar. It's perfect for helping you meet your protein needs during your soft-foods stage.

4½ cups Savory Chicken Broth (page 144) or store-bought chicken broth

1 cup sliced carrots

1 (8-ounce) can bamboo shoots, drained

1 (8-ounce) can water chestnuts, drained

1 (4-ounce) can sliced mushrooms, drained

¼ cup rice vinegar

4 teaspoons low-sodium soy sauce or coconut aminos

1 teaspoon coconut sugar

½ teaspoon red pepper flakes

2 tablespoons arrowroot starch

2 tablespoons water

8 ounces pork shoulder or loin, sliced

4 to 6 ounces firm tofu, drained and cubed

Sliced scallions, for topping

1. In a 6-quart slow cooker, combine the broth, carrots, bamboo shoots, water chestnuts, mushrooms, vinegar, soy sauce, sugar, and red pepper flakes. Cover and cook on low for 7 hours.

2. In a small bowl, mix together the arrowroot starch and water to make a slurry.

3. Remove the slow cooker lid and add the slurry, pork, and tofu. Cover, increase the heat to high, and cook for an additional 30 minutes.

4. Turn off the slow cooker. Garnish with scallions, and serve the soup warm. Refrigerate leftovers for up to 5 days, or freeze for up to 1 month.

> TIP
>
> Can't find arrowroot starch? Swap it out for the same amount of cornstarch.

SERVING RECOMMENDATIONS

Soft Foods: ½ cup
General Foods: 1 cup

Per serving: Calories: 149; Protein: 10g; Fat: 6g; Carbohydrates: 14g; Fiber: 2g; Sugar: 4g; Sodium: 150mg

(S) (G)

Hearty Beef and Barley Stew

Prep time: 15 minutes
Cook time: 8 hours on low
SERVES 8 TO 10

Whole-grain barley is rich in magnesium, potassium, B vitamins, and fiber, making it an excellent addition to any stew or side dish. The texture of this Moroccan-inspired stew is perfect for your healing stomach, particularly in the soft-foods stage. You'll also meet your protein and vegetable goals, and you can boost your protein even more with a dollop of Greek yogurt on top.

2 pounds stew beef, cut into bite-size cubes

½ teaspoon sea salt, plus more for seasoning

½ teaspoon ground black pepper, plus more for seasoning

3 tablespoons extra-virgin olive oil

1 cup sliced carrots

1 large onion, diced

2 large white potatoes (skin on), cut into bite-size pieces

4 teaspoons minced garlic

6 cups beef broth

1½ cups pearled barley

2 teaspoons dried thyme

½ teaspoon dried rosemary

¼ cup tomato paste

1 tablespoon Worcestershire sauce

1 or 2 bay leaves

1 to 1¼ cups plain 2 percent Greek yogurt, for topping (optional)

Chopped fresh parsley, for topping (optional)

1. Season the beef with salt and black pepper.

2. Coat the bottom of a 6-quart slow cooker with the olive oil.

3. Set the heat to high. Add the beef and cook, stirring occasionally, for 3 to 4 minutes.

4. Add the carrots, onion, potatoes, garlic, broth, barley, thyme, rosemary, tomato paste, Worcestershire sauce, salt, black pepper, and bay leaf. Mix well. Cover, reduce the heat to low, and cook for 8 hours.

5. Turn off the slow cooker. Discard the bay leaf. Top with 2 tablespoons of Greek yogurt per serving (if using) and parsley (if using). Serve the stew warm.

6. Refrigerate leftovers for up to 1 week, or freeze for up to 2 months.

This can be made gluten-free by using brown or white rice in place of the barley and making sure to use broth that is labeled gluten-free.

SERVING RECOMMENDATIONS

Soft Foods: ½ cup
General Foods: 1 cup

Per serving: Calories: 406; Protein: 31g; Fat: 10g; Carbohydrates: 50g; Fiber: 9g; Sugar: 4g; Sodium: 239mg

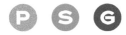

Comforting Chicken and Rice Soup

Prep time: 15 minutes
Cook time: 7 hours on low
SERVES 6 TO 8

This comfort-food staple will deliver on fiber, essential minerals, protein, B vitamins, and vegetables. With tender chicken breasts and a creamy base, it's sure to satisfy your comfort-food cravings while also nourishing your healing stomach.

1 cup wild rice, rinsed and drained

1½ pounds boneless, skinless chicken breasts

2 cups sliced carrots

1 cup sliced celery

1 small yellow onion, diced

4 teaspoons minced garlic

1 teaspoon dried rosemary

1 teaspoon dried thyme

2 teaspoons sea salt

½ teaspoon ground black pepper

1 or 2 bay leaves

6 cups Savory Chicken Broth (page 144) or store-bought chicken broth

3 tablespoons extra-virgin olive oil

2 cups unsweetened almond or oat milk

½ cup whole-wheat flour

Chopped fresh parsley, fresh thyme, or freshly squeezed lemon or lime juice, for topping (optional)

1. In a 6-quart slow cooker, combine the rice, chicken, carrots, celery, onion, garlic, rosemary, thyme, salt, black pepper, bay leaf, and broth. Cover and cook on low for 7 hours, until the chicken has cooked through and the vegetables are soft.

2. Remove the lid and remove the chicken. Shred using 2 forks. Return the meat to the slow cooker and stir.

3. In a medium bowl, whisk together the olive oil, milk, and flour until any lumps have dissolved and the mixture is thick and creamy. Pour into the slow cooker and mix well.

4. Turn off the slow cooker. Discard the bay leaf. Serve the soup warm, garnished with parsley, thyme, or lemon juice (if using).

5. Refrigerate leftovers for up to 1 week, or freeze for up to 2 months.

To make this recipe for your puree recovery stage, transfer one serving at a time to a blender or food processor and puree until smooth.

Pureed Foods: ¼–½ cup
Soft Foods: ½ cup
General Foods: 1 cup

Per serving: Calories: 352; Protein: 32g; Fat: 10g; Carbohydrates: 35g; Fiber: 5g; Sugar: 4g; Sodium: 509mg

(S) (G)

Easy Seafood Stew

Prep time: 15 minutes
Cook time: 6 hours on low and 1 hour on high
SERVES 6 TO 8

If you love fish and seafood, this easy stew may become your new go-to! It will provide you with all the protein, fiber, and fluid you need to stay full and hydrated while also being gentle on your stomach. Switch up the types of fish and seafood you use each time you make this for a fun twist. Serve this with ½ slice of bread or 3 crackers of your choice.

1 (28-ounce) can crushed tomatoes

3 cups Savory Vegetable Broth (page 146) or store-bought vegetable broth

1 (8-ounce) can clam juice

¼ cup white-wine vinegar

¼ cup water

4 teaspoons minced garlic

3½ cups chopped and peeled baby potatoes

1 small yellow onion, diced

1 teaspoon dried basil

1 teaspoon dried cilantro

1 teaspoon dried thyme

1 teaspoon sea salt

½ teaspoon ground black pepper

¼ teaspoon red pepper flakes

2 pounds frozen seafood mix, thawed

1. In a 6-quart slow cooker, combine the tomatoes, broth, clam juice, vinegar, water, garlic, potatoes, onion, basil, cilantro, thyme, salt, black pepper, and red pepper flakes. Cover and cook on low for 6 hours, until the potatoes are very tender.

2. Remove the lid and stir in the thawed seafood mix. Cover, increase the heat to high, and cook for an additional 30 minutes to 1 hour, until the seafood has cooked through.

3. Turn off the slow cooker. Serve the stew warm. Refrigerate leftovers for up to 5 days, or freeze for up to 1 month.

SERVING RECOMMENDATIONS

Soft Foods: ½ cup
General Foods: 1 cup

Per serving: Calories: 282; Protein: 30g; Fat: 6g; Carbohydrates: 27g; Fiber: 5g; Sugar: 6g; Sodium: 851mg

Hearty Beanless Chili

Prep time: 15 minutes
Cook time: 3 minutes on high and 6 hours on low
SERVES 6 TO 8

Boost your protein intake and reduce chances of uncomfortable gas with this beanless chili! It will warm you up and fill you up with plenty of protein, B vitamins, vegetables, and fiber. This recipe is particularly great if you struggle to digest beans without excess gas but still enjoy chili flavors. Enjoy during your soft-foods stage and beyond.

1 tablespoon extra-virgin olive oil

1 pound 85 percent lean ground beef

1 pound ground pork

1 (28-ounce) can tomato sauce

1 (28-ounce) can crushed tomatoes

1 (6-ounce) can tomato paste

1 medium yellow onion, diced

1 large yellow or orange bell pepper, cored and diced

3 tablespoons minced garlic

1 cup beef broth

2 tablespoons chili powder

1 teaspoon cayenne pepper

½ teaspoon sea salt

½ teaspoon ground black pepper

Chopped fresh cilantro, sliced scallions, or sliced avocado, for topping (optional)

¾ to 1 cup sour cream, for topping (optional)

¾ to 1 cup guacamole, for topping (optional)

1. Coat the bottom of a 6-quart slow cooker with the olive oil.

2. Set the heat to high. Add the beef and pork. Cook, stirring occasionally, for 2 to 3 minutes.

3. Add the tomato sauce, crushed tomatoes, tomato paste, onion, bell pepper, garlic, broth, chili powder, cayenne, salt, and black pepper. Stir. Cover, reduce the heat to low, and cook for 6 hours, until the pork has cooked through and the vegetables are soft.

4. Turn off the slow cooker. Top with cilantro, scallions, or avocado (if using); 2 tablespoons of sour cream per serving (if using); or 2 tablespoons of guacamole per serving (if using). Do not add scallions if you are at the soft-foods stage. Serve the chili warm.

5. Refrigerate leftovers for up to 1 week, or freeze for up to 2 months.

CONTINUED →

Hearty Beanless Chili CONTINUED

TIP

For a leaner option, replace the ground beef and pork with chicken, turkey, or a combination of both.

SERVING RECOMMENDATIONS

Soft Foods: ½ cup
General Foods: 1 cup

Per serving: Calories: 489; Protein: 32g; Fat: 31g; Carbohydrates: 24g; Fiber: 8g; Sugar: 13g; Sodium: 460mg

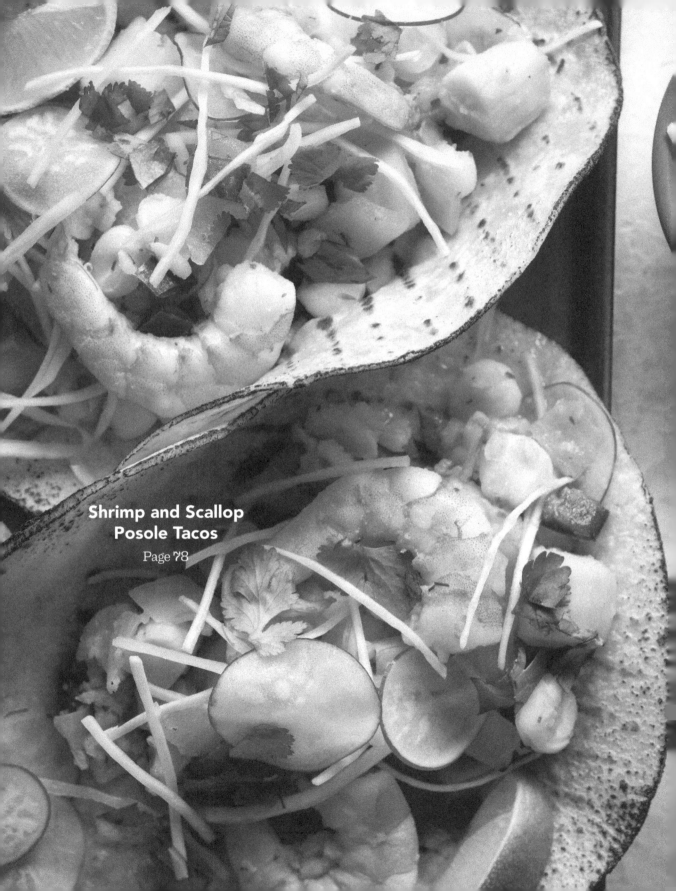

**Shrimp and Scallop
Posole Tacos**

Page 78

5

Seafood & Vegetarian

 LIQUIDS   SOFT FOODS   PUREED FOODS   Ⓖ GENERAL FOODS FOR LIFE

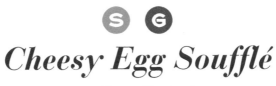

Cheesy Egg Soufflé

Prep time: 15 minutes
Cook time: 5 to 6 hours on low
SERVES 6

Egg soufflés can feel intimidating to make, but this recipe makes it so easy. And it's simply delicious! The texture and protein content make it a perfect vegetarian dish for your healing stomach, particularly during your soft-foods stage. This also reheats well in the microwave.

Nonstick cooking spray, for coating the slow cooker

1 loaf fresh whole-wheat bread, crusts removed

1 cup shredded sharp Cheddar cheese, divided

1 cup shredded mozzarella cheese, divided

1 cup shredded Monterey Jack cheese, divided

4 tablespoons (½ stick) butter, at room temperature, divided

6 large eggs

1 cup 2 percent milk

1 cup half-and-half

2 teaspoons chopped fresh parsley

½ teaspoon sea salt

1. Coat the bottom of a 6-quart slow cooker with cooking spray.

2. Rip apart the bread and put half on the bottom of the slow cooker, followed, in order, by ½ cup of Cheddar cheese, ½ cup of mozzarella cheese, and ½ cup of Monterey Jack cheese.

3. Spread or arrange small dollops of butter over the cheese, 2 tablespoons total.

4. Repeat the layering process with the remaining bread, ½ cup of Cheddar cheese, ½ cup of mozzarella cheese, ½ cup of Monterey Jack cheese, and 2 tablespoons of butter.

5. In a large bowl, whisk together the eggs, milk, half-and-half, parsley, and salt.

6. Pour the egg mixture over the bread and cheese. Cover and cook on low for 5 to 6 hours, until the eggs have set.

7. Turn off the slow cooker. Serve the soufflé warm.

8. Refrigerate leftovers for up to 5 days, or freeze for up to 1 month.

Serve with ¼ cup of fresh fruit or ¼ cup of sliced avocado on the side.

TIP

Use any combination of cheeses you prefer, including goat, feta, Colby, Swiss, etc.

SERVING RECOMMENDATIONS

Soft Foods: ½ cup
General Foods: 1 cup

Per serving: Calories: 667; Protein: 35g; Fat: 38g; Carbohydrates: 47g; Fiber: 6g; Sugar: 9g; Sodium: 971mg

Shrimp and Scallop Posole Tacos

Prep time: 15 minutes
Cook time: 5 hours 20 minutes on low
SERVES 4

Posole is a Latin American soup or stew made with hominy, or whole dried field corn, and a variety of proteins. Popular toppings include lime, cilantro, cabbage, and radishes, as included in this recipe. Slow-cooking allows for the full flavors to develop while you to step away. When you come back, you'll have a delicious lunch or dinner.

2 cups Savory Vegetable Broth (page 146) or store-bought vegetable broth

2 cups canned white hominy, drained and rinsed

2 medium yellow onions, diced

1 or 2 poblano chiles (depending on your desired spice level), cored and diced

3 tablespoons ground cumin

1 tablespoon minced garlic

4 teaspoons dried oregano

1½ pounds frozen deveined peeled shrimp, thawed

1½ pounds frozen scallops, thawed

½ teaspoon sea salt

8 to 10 corn tortillas

Shredded cabbage, sliced radishes, chopped fresh cilantro, lime juice, or extra-virgin olive oil, for topping (optional)

1. In a 6-quart slow cooker, combine the broth, hominy, onions, chiles, cumin, garlic, and oregano. Cover and cook on low for 5 hours, until the vegetables are soft.

2. Remove the lid and add the shrimp and scallops. Replace the lid and cook for an additional 15 to 20 minutes, until the shrimp are pink and the scallops are opaque.

3. Turn off the slow cooker. Stir in the salt.

4. Spoon about ¼ cup of the cooked posole into a corn tortilla for each serving.

5. Top with shredded cabbage, sliced radishes, chopped cilantro, lime juice, or olive oil (if using). Serve the tacos warm.

6. Refrigerate leftovers for up to 5 days, or freeze for up to 1 month.

Modify the spice level by altering the amount of chiles, cumin, garlic, and oregano.

SERVING RECOMMENDATIONS

Soft Foods: ¼ cup in 1 corn tortilla
General Foods: ½ cup split between 2 corn tortillas

Per serving: Calories: 241; Protein: 30g; Fat: 2g; Carbohydrates: 25g; Fiber: 3g; Sugar: 2g; Sodium: 658mg

Salmon, Pasta, and Vegetable Bake

Prep time: 15 minutes
Cook time: 3 minutes on high and 5 to 6 hours on low
SERVES 6 TO 8

Get your protein, vegetables, B vitamins, omega-3s, and fiber all in one dish! Cooking pasta in the slow cooker removes the need to stand over a pot on the stove until the pasta has finished cooking. Simply layer the ingredients, step away, and let it cook.

1 tablespoon extra-virgin olive oil

1 tablespoon minced garlic

1 pound cremini mushrooms, sliced

1 medium yellow onion, diced

1 red bell pepper, cored and diced

6 cups baby spinach (about 5 ounces)

1 (15-ounce) container ricotta cheese

1 large egg

2 cups shredded mozzarella cheese, divided

½ cup grated Parmesan cheese, divided

2 (24-ounce) jars no-sugar-added red pasta sauce of your choice, divided

1 pound whole-grain penne, divided

1 pound wild-caught salmon fillets (3 or 4 fillets)

½ lemon

Sea salt

Ground black pepper

1. In a 6-quart slow cooker, combine the olive oil, garlic, mushrooms, onion, and bell pepper. Cook on high for 2 to 3 minutes, until warm.

2. Add the spinach 1 cup at a time, allowing it to wilt a bit in between additions. Stir well.

3. In a large bowl, mix together the ricotta cheese, egg, 1 cup of mozzarella cheese, and ¼ cup of Parmesan cheese.

4. Transfer half of the vegetable mixture from the slow cooker to a separate large bowl.

5. Pour 1 cup of pasta sauce over the vegetables remaining in the slow cooker.

6. Arrange half of the penne in a layer over the sauce, followed, in order, by 2 cups of pasta sauce, half of the ricotta mixture, and about half of the vegetable mixture that you transferred to the bowl. Repeat this layering step once more. Cover and cook on low for 4 to 5 hours, until the noodles are cooked and the vegetables are soft.

7. Remove the lid and sprinkle the remaining 1 cup of mozzarella cheese and ¼ cup of Parmesan cheese over the pasta and vegetables.

8. Lay the salmon fillets flat on top of the cheese, and squeeze the lemon lightly over the top of the fillets.

9. Pour the remaining 1 cup of pasta sauce over the salmon.

10. Replace the lid and cook for an additional 30 minutes to 1 hour, until the salmon is cooked through.

11. Turn off the slow cooker. Season with salt and pepper to taste and serve the pasta bake warm.

12. Refrigerate leftovers for up to 5 days, or freeze for up to 1 month.

TIP

You can remove the salmon fillets when they are done cooking and shred them using a fork before adding them back to the pasta.

SERVING RECOMMENDATIONS

Soft Foods: ½ cup
General Foods: 1 cup

Per serving: Calories: 752; Protein: 52g; Fat: 29g; Carbohydrates: 77g; Fiber: 13g; Sugar: 10g; Sodium: 575mg

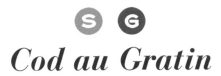

Cod au Gratin

Prep time: 15 to 20 minutes
Cook time: 4 minutes on high and 6 hours on low
SERVES 6 TO 8

"Au gratin" is a French dish typically encompassing potatoes, cheese, milk, and spices. With this recipe, I added the cod as a lean protein to support healthy blood sugar and weight management.

Nonstick cooking spray, for coating the slow cooker

4 tablespoons (½ stick) butter

¼ cup whole-wheat flour

2½ cups 2 percent milk

2 teaspoons garlic powder

½ teaspoon sea salt

½ teaspoon ground black pepper

1½ cups shredded sharp Cheddar cheese

1½ cups grated Parmesan cheese, divided

2 pounds white potatoes, peeled and cut into ½-inch-thick slices

1 pound wild-caught cod (3 or 4 large fillets)

1 lemon

1 teaspoon chopped fresh thyme, plus more for topping

1 teaspoon dried rosemary, plus more for topping

1. Generously coat the bottom and sides of a 6-quart slow cooker with cooking spray.

2. Add the butter and melt on high.

3. Add the flour and milk. Whisk for 3 to 4 minutes, until simmering and thickened.

4. Mix in the garlic powder, salt, and black pepper.

5. Turn off the slow cooker. Whisk in the Cheddar cheese and ¼ cup of Parmesan cheese. Leaving a thin layer of the cheese sauce in the bottom of the slow cooker, transfer the remaining sauce to a large bowl.

6. In the slow cooker, arrange a layer of potatoes on top of the cheese sauce, followed by one-quarter of the cheese sauce from the bowl and a thin sprinkling of Parmesan cheese. Repeat with the remaining potatoes, cheese sauce, and Parmesan cheese (making sure Parmesan is the last layer at the end). Cover and cook on low for 5 hours, until the potatoes are tender.

7. Remove the lid and arrange the cod in a single layer on top of the potato and cheese layers.

8. Squeeze the lemon lightly over the top of the cod, and top with the thyme and rosemary. Replace the lid and cook for an additional 30 minutes to 1 hour, until the cod has cooked through.

9. Turn off the slow cooker. Garnish with additional lemon juice, thyme, and rosemary. Serve the gratin warm.

10. Refrigerate leftovers for up to 5 days, or freeze for up to 1 month.

SERVING RECOMMENDATIONS

Soft Foods: ½ cup
General Foods: 1 cup

Per serving: Calories: 529; Protein: 33g; Fat: 27g; Carbohydrates: 40g; Fiber: 4g; Sugar: 7g; Sodium: 877mg

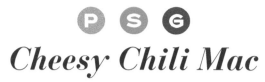

Cheesy Chili Mac

Prep time: 15 minutes
Cook time: 3 minutes on high and 7 hours 40 minutes on low
SERVES 8 TO 10

This easy cheesy meal may just become your next family favorite! With a blend of whole grains, legumes, and shredded cheese, you'll meet your protein goal while also boosting your fiber intake. The spices add some heat, while the tomatoes and onion lend texture.

Nonstick cooking spray, for coating the slow cooker

5 tablespoons minced garlic

3 (15-ounce) cans beans of your choice (pinto, kidney, black, navy, etc.)

3 cups canned diced tomatoes, drained

1 small yellow onion, diced

4 cups Savory Vegetable Broth (page 146) or store-bought vegetable broth

½ teaspoon sea salt

½ teaspoon ground black pepper

2 teaspoons chili powder

1 teaspoon paprika

2 tablespoons ground cumin

½ teaspoon cayenne pepper

8 ounces whole-grain macaroni

8 ounces shredded mild Cheddar cheese

8 ounces shredded Colby-Jack cheese

1. Generously coat the bottom and sides of a 6-quart slow cooker with cooking spray.

2. Set the heat to high. Add the garlic and cook for 2 to 3 minutes, until fragrant.

3. Mix in the beans, tomatoes, onion, broth, salt, black pepper, chili powder, paprika, cumin, and cayenne. Cover, reduce the heat to low, and cook for 7 hours, until the beans are easily mashed.

4. Remove the lid and add the macaroni. Mix well. Replace the lid and cook for an additional 20 to 30 minutes, until the macaroni is soft.

5. Remove the lid and stir in the Cheddar cheese and Colby-Jack cheese. Replace the lid and cook for an additional 5 to 10 minutes, until the cheese has begun to melt.

6. Turn off the slow cooker. Serve the chili mac warm.

7. Refrigerate leftovers for up to 1 week, or freeze for up to 3 months.

To make this recipe for your puree recovery stage, simply use an immersion blender to puree after cooking.

SERVING RECOMMENDATIONS

Pureed Foods: ¼-½ cup
Soft Foods: ½ cup
General Foods: 1 cup

Per serving: Calories: 483; Protein: 28g; Fat: 20g; Carbohydrates: 51g; Fiber: 12g; Sugar: 3g; Sodium: 456mg

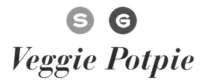

Veggie Potpie

Prep time: 15 minutes
Cook time: 6 hours 45 minutes on low
SERVES 6

A true comfort-food classic, this potpie is extra easy. Lentils uniquely bolster the protein content, while the variety of vegetables gives this potpie a strong lead in the fiber department. Perfect for your soft-foods stage of recovery.

1 tablespoon extra-virgin olive oil

3 cups Savory Vegetable Broth (page 146) or store-bought vegetable broth, divided

2 tablespoons cornstarch

1 pound white potatoes, peeled and diced

1 medium white or yellow onion, diced

1½ cups sliced carrots

1 cup sliced celery

8 ounces cremini mushrooms, stemmed and sliced

2 teaspoons minced garlic

1 teaspoon sea salt

½ teaspoon ground black pepper

1 teaspoon dried thyme

1 or 2 bay leaves

1 cup dried green lentils

1 cup frozen corn kernels

¼ cup sliced scallions, both white and green parts

¾ cup 2 percent milk

1 tablespoon white-wine vinegar or lemon juice

1 (16.3-ounce) container flaky biscuit dough (such as Pillsbury Grands! Southern Homestyle), cut into small wedges

1. Coat the bottom of a 6-quart slow cooker with the olive oil.

2. In a medium bowl, whisk together 1½ cups of broth and the cornstarch.

3. To the slow cooker, add the potatoes, onion, carrots, celery, mushrooms, garlic, salt, black pepper, thyme, bay leaf, and lentils.

4. Pour the broth and cornstarch mixture and the remaining 1½ cups of broth over the vegetables. Mix well. Cover and cook on low for 6 hours, until the vegetables and lentils are tender.

5. Remove the lid and stir in the corn, scallions, milk, vinegar, and biscuit dough. Replace the lid and cook for an additional 45 minutes, until the biscuit wedges have cooked through.

6. Turn off the slow cooker. Discard the bay leaf. Serve the potpie warm.

7. Refrigerate leftovers for up to 1 week, or freeze for up to 1 month.

TIP

Substitute white beans or edamame for the lentils for a variety of protein- and fiber-rich options.

SERVING RECOMMENDATIONS

Soft Foods: ½ cup
General Foods: 1 cup

Per serving: Calories: 498; Protein: 17g; Fat: 11g; Carbohydrates: 85g; Fiber: 8g; Sugar: 12g; Sodium: 904mg

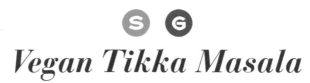

Vegan Tikka Masala

Prep time: 15 minutes
Cook time: 8 hours 30 minutes on low
SERVES 6

Chicken tikka masala was made popular by Bengali chefs in 1970s Britain. This hot and spicy vegan version is a protein-rich, plant-based alternative to the original. Its soft and tender texture is also perfect for your soft-foods stage of recovery. This dish reheats well in the microwave.

2 tablespoons olive oil

4 (15-ounce) cans chickpeas, drained and rinsed

1 large yellow onion, chopped

5 teaspoons minced garlic

2 tablespoons grated fresh ginger

1 (15-ounce) can tomato sauce

2 teaspoons sea salt

½ teaspoon ground black pepper

1 teaspoon ground coriander

1 teaspoon ground turmeric

¼ teaspoon ground cinnamon

½ teaspoon cayenne pepper

2 teaspoons ground cumin

2 teaspoons paprika

1 tablespoon garam masala

1 cup full-fat canned coconut milk

2 tablespoons cornstarch

1 tablespoon lemon juice

Chopped fresh cilantro, for topping

1½ cups cooked brown or basmati rice

1. Coat the bottom of a 6-quart slow cooker with the olive oil.

2. Add the chickpeas, onion, garlic, ginger, tomato sauce, salt, black pepper, coriander, turmeric, cinnamon, cayenne, cumin, paprika, and garam masala. Mix well so the chickpeas are well coated. Cover and cook on low for 8 hours, until the chickpeas are tender.

3. In a small bowl, whisk together the coconut milk and cornstarch to make a slurry.

4. Remove the slow cooker lid and stir in the slurry. Replace the lid and cook for an additional 30 minutes, until the gravy has thickened.

5. Turn off the slow cooker. Stir in the lemon juice, and garnish with the cilantro.

6. Serve the tikka masala over ¼ cup of rice per serving.

7. Refrigerate leftovers for up to 1 week, or freeze for up to 2 months.

If you'd like a grain-free option, substitute cauliflower rice for the rice.

SERVING RECOMMENDATIONS

Soft Foods: ½ cup
General Foods: 1 cup

Per serving: Calories: 481; Protein: 18g; Fat: 18g; Carbohydrates: 67g; Fiber: 16g; Sugar: 11g; Sodium: 492mg

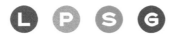

Creamy Homemade Greek Yogurt

Prep time: 10 minutes
Cook time: 3 hours 30 minutes on low, plus 12 hours to rest
SERVES 6

This protein- and calcium-rich food can be blended with sweet and savory toppings alike. It's also perfect for any stage of your recovery. Given that, it may be cheaper to make your own than to purchase store brands. Meet your protein needs quickly and for any meal. This is best served chilled.

1 gallon 2 percent or whole milk (do not use ultrapasteurized)

1 cup plain 2 percent or 4 percent yogurt

Fresh honey, chopped fresh fruit, nut butter, or coconut flakes, for topping (optional; see Tip)

1. Pour the milk into a 6-quart slow cooker. Cover and cook on low for 3 to 3½ hours, until hot.

2. Turn off the slow cooker. Let the milk sit covered for an additional 3 hours.

3. Transfer 3 cups of the warm milk to a large bowl. Whisk in the yogurt.

4. Add the milk and yogurt mixture to the slow cooker and whisk well. Replace the lid and wrap a towel around the entire slow cooker. Let the yogurt mixture sit for 8 hours, until the texture looks like plain yogurt.

5. To make a thick Greek yogurt, place a colander over a large bowl or sink and layer it with paper towels. Spoon the yogurt into the colander to drain for about 1 hour, until thick and creamy. Chill before serving.

6. Serve the yogurt cold with fresh honey, fresh fruit, nut butter, or coconut flakes (if using), depending on which recovery stage you are in (see Tip on page 91).

7. Refrigerate leftovers for up to 1 week, or freeze for up to 2 months.

During your liquids and pureed-foods recovery stages, serve with honey only. For your soft-foods and general-foods stages, serve with berries or banana and nut butter. If you are in the general-foods stage, you can also serve with coconut flakes.

SERVING RECOMMENDATIONS

Liquids: ¼–½ cup
Pureed Foods: ¼–½ cup
Soft Foods: ½ cup
General Foods: 1 cup

Per serving: Calories: 351; Protein: 24g; Fat: 14g; Carbohydrates: 34g; Fiber: 0g; Sugar: 36g; Sodium: 334mg

Very Veggie Lasagna

Prep time: 15 minutes
Cook time: 4 minutes on high and
5 hours 30 minutes on low, plus 1 hour to rest
SERVES 6 TO 8

Comforting and rich in protein, fiber, and vegetables, this lasagna will likely become a favorite! This recipe is also easily modifiable to your preferences for texture and flavor since you can mix and match the vegetables and cheeses and cook longer for a softer noodle texture. Given this flexibility, it's perfect for your soft-foods stage of recovery.

2 tablespoons extra-virgin olive oil

1 pound cremini mushrooms, chopped

1 medium yellow onion, chopped

1 cup finely chopped peeled zucchini or yellow squash

½ teaspoon sea salt

3 to 4½ cups red pasta sauce (depending on how saucy you want it to be), divided

8 to 10 thick lasagna noodles

1 (24-ounce) container 2 percent small-curd cottage cheese, divided

2 cups shredded mozzarella or provolone cheese, divided

2 (10-ounce) bags frozen chopped spinach, divided

1 teaspoon Italian seasoning

Grated Parmesan, pesto, or chopped fresh parsley, for topping (optional)

1. Coat the bottom of a 6-quart slow cooker with the olive oil.

2. Set the heat to high. Add the mushrooms, onion, zucchini, and salt. Cook, stirring every minute or so, for 3 to 4 minutes, until the vegetables begin to sizzle. Transfer to a large bowl.

3. Reduce the heat to low. Pour half of the pasta sauce into the bottom of the slow cooker in an even layer.

4. Place 2 whole lasagna noodles on top of the sauce, and break a third in half to fill in the sides if needed.

5. Spread one-third of the cottage cheese on top of noodles, followed by 1 cup of the vegetable mixture, ²/³ cup of mozzarella cheese, and a thin layer of frozen spinach.

6. Repeat with the remaining cottage cheese, vegetable mixture, and frozen spinach.

7. Top with the remaining tomato sauce, and sprinkle the Italian seasoning over the top.

8. Cover and cook on low for 5 hours, until the noodles are cooked and the lasagna is heated through.

9. Remove the lid and sprinkle the remaining 1⅓ cups of mozzarella cheese over the top. Replace the lid and cook for an additional 30 minutes, until the cheese has melted and is bubbly.

10. Turn off the slow cooker. Let the lasagna sit for 1 hour before serving. This will ensure a firmer texture. If you prefer a thinner, soup-like lasagna, serve immediately.

11. Top with grated Parmesan, pesto, or parsley (if using). Serve the lasagna warm.

12. Refrigerate leftovers for up to 1 week, or freeze for up to 2 months.

TIP

Cook for an additional hour for softer noodles (but still allow the lasagna to sit for 1 hour after cooking).

SERVING RECOMMENDATIONS

Soft Foods: ½ cup
General Foods: 1 cup

Per serving: Calories: 487; Protein: 33g; Fat: 19g; Carbohydrates: 49g; Fiber: 7g; Sugar: 12g; Sodium: 835mg

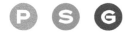

Meatless Veggie Chili

Prep time: 15 minutes
Cook time: 4 minutes on high and 7 to 8 hours on low
SERVES 8 TO 10

This super easy plant-based chili provides you with the protein and fiber you need to fill up and stay full, all without meat or poultry. Beans deliver on the protein front, while both the beans and vegetables provide fiber. This meal is appropriate for the soft-foods stage and is easily reheated in the microwave or on the stovetop.

2 tablespoons extra-virgin olive oil

1 large yellow onion, chopped

2 cups chopped celery, chopped

1 yellow bell pepper, cored and chopped

1 orange bell pepper, cored and chopped

1 red bell pepper, cored and chopped

½ teaspoon sea salt, plus more for seasoning

4 (28-ounce) cans crushed tomatoes

2 (15-ounce) cans kidney beans, drained and rinsed

1 (15-ounce) can cannellini beans, drained and rinsed

1 (15-ounce) can black beans, drained and rinsed

4 teaspoons minced garlic

2 to 3 teaspoons chili powder (more if you want it spicier)

3 to 4 tablespoons ground cumin

2 teaspoons dried oregano

Ground black pepper

Sliced avocado, chopped fresh cilantro, or sliced scallions, for topping (optional)

1 to 1¼ cups shredded Cheddar or Monterey Jack cheese, for topping (optional)

1 to 1¼ cups guacamole, for topping (optional)

1 to 1¼ cups sour cream, for topping (optional)

1. Coat the bottom of a 6-quart slow cooker with the olive oil.

2. Set the heat to high. Add the onion, celery, yellow bell pepper, orange bell pepper, red bell pepper, and salt. Cook, stirring every minute or so, for 3 to 4 minutes, until the vegetables start to sizzle.

3. Reduce the heat to low. Add the tomatoes, kidney beans, cannellini beans, black beans, garlic, chili powder, cumin, and oregano. Season with salt and black pepper. Cover and cook on low for 7 to 8 hours, until the vegetables are soft and the beans are easily mashed.

4. Turn off the slow cooker. Top with any combination of avocado, cilantro, or scallions (if using); 2 tablespoons of cheese per serving (if using); 2 tablespoons of guacamole per serving (if using); or 2 tablespoons of sour cream per serving (if using). Do not add the cilantro or scallions if you are at the pureed-foods stage, and avoid scallions at the soft-foods stage. Serve the chili warm.

5. Refrigerate leftovers for up to 1 week, or freeze for up to 3 months.

TIP

To make this recipe for your puree recovery stage, simply use an immersion blender to puree after cooking.

SERVING RECOMMENDATIONS

Pureed Foods: ¼–½ cup
Soft Foods: ½ cup
General Foods: 1 cup

Per serving: Calories: 370; Protein: 19g; Fat: 6g; Carbohydrates: 69g; Fiber: 20g; Sugar: 20g; Sodium: 886mg

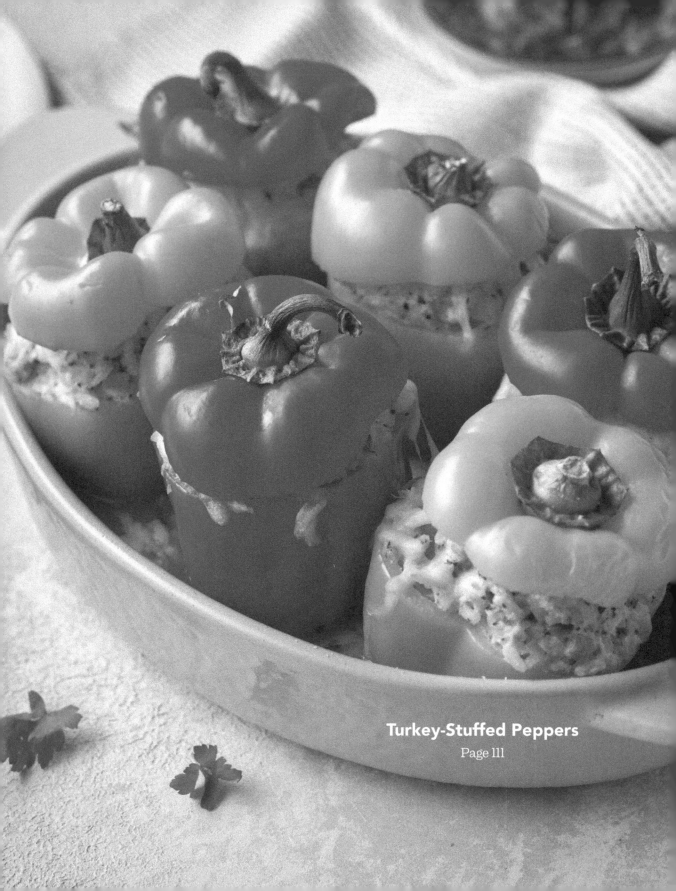

Turkey-Stuffed Peppers

Page 111

6

Poultry & Meat

Ⓛ LIQUIDS Ⓢ SOFT FOODS Ⓟ PUREED FOODS Ⓖ GENERAL FOODS FOR LIFE

Cheesy Chicken and Rice

Prep time: 15 minutes
Cook time: 6 hours 30 minutes on low
SERVES 8

Meet your protein and fiber needs with this easy, filling, and comforting meal. Throw in all the ingredients except for the cheese and parsley and walk away. Its soft texture is perfect for your soft-foods healing stage, and if needed, you can chop the chicken extra small to make digestion even easier. This is easy to reheat in the microwave or on the stove.

2 tablespoons extra-virgin olive oil

3 large boneless, skinless chicken breasts, chopped into bite-size pieces

2 teaspoons minced garlic

1½ teaspoons sea salt

1 teaspoon ground black pepper

1 small white onion, finely chopped

4½ cups Savory Chicken Broth (page 144) or store-bought chicken broth

2 cups sour cream or plain Greek yogurt

2¼ cups wild rice

2 cups diced carrots

2 cups shredded Cheddar, Monterey Jack, or Colby-Jack cheese

Chopped fresh parsley, for topping

1 cup grated Parmesan cheese

1. Coat the bottom of a 6-quart slow cooker with the olive oil.

2. Add the chicken, garlic, salt, black pepper, onion, broth, sour cream, rice, and carrots. Stir. Cover and cook on low for 6 hours, until the chicken has cooked through.

3. Remove the lid and stir in the Cheddar cheese. Replace the lid and cook for an additional 30 minutes, until the cheese has melted.

4. Turn off the slow cooker. Top with parsley and 2 tablespoons of Parmesan cheese per serving. Serve the chicken and rice warm.

5. Refrigerate leftovers for up to 5 days, or freeze for up to 2 months.

You can use long-grain brown rice instead of wild if you prefer. You can also use peas instead of carrots—or 1 cup of each. If you need more moisture, simply add another ½ to 1 cup of chicken broth.

SERVING RECOMMENDATIONS

Soft Foods: ½ cup
General Foods: 1 cup

Per serving: Calories: 510; Protein: 29g; Fat: 27g; Carbohydrates: 40g; Fiber: 4g; Sugar: 5g; Sodium: 501mg

Garlic-Honey Chicken and Carrots

Prep time: 15 minutes
Cook time: 7 hours 45 minutes on low
SERVES 8 TO 10

This sweet and tangy entrée is perfect for those nights when you're craving something a little sweet. Satisfy your cravings while also meeting your protein, iron, B vitamin, and fiber needs. The tanginess in this recipe is also easily modifiable by simply adjusting the amount of vinegar you use. Enjoy these rich flavors during your soft-foods healing stage!

1 cup low-sodium soy sauce or coconut aminos

¾ cup honey

2 teaspoons minced garlic

¼ cup tomato paste

2 to 3 tablespoons apple cider vinegar

2 tablespoons extra-virgin olive oil

5 boneless, skinless chicken breasts

3 cups baby carrots

1 small white onion, chopped

1 teaspoon sea salt

1 teaspoon ground black pepper

20 ounces fresh green beans, trimmed (optional)

2 tablespoons chopped fresh parsley, for topping

1. In a large bowl, whisk together the soy sauce, honey, garlic, tomato paste, and vinegar.

2. Coat the bottom of a 6-quart slow cooker with the olive oil.

3. Add the chicken, carrots, onion, salt, black pepper, and soy sauce mixture. Mix well. Cover and cook on low for 7 hours, until the chicken has cooked through.

4. Remove the lid and add the green beans (if using). Mix well. Replace the lid and cook for an additional 30 to 45 minutes, until the green beans are tender.

5. Turn off the slow cooker. Sprinkle the parsley over the top, and serve warm.

6. Refrigerate leftovers for up to 5 days, or freeze for up to 3 months.

SERVING RECOMMENDATIONS

Soft Foods: ½ cup
General Foods: 1 cup

Per serving: Calories: 326; Protein: 29g; Fat: 7g; Carbohydrates: 40g; Fiber: 4g; Sugar: 32g; Sodium: 1,385mg

Chicken Cacciatore

Prep time: 15 minutes
Cook time: 6 hours 30 minutes on low
SERVES 8 TO 10

This classic Italian dish could not be easier! Simply add the ingredients in two steps and let it cook. I've found the slow cooker to be the simplest way to cook a protein and a pasta together, without all the separate pots and pans. This dish is perfect for your soft-foods stage and will provide protein, iron, B vitamins, and fiber.

3 tablespoons extra-virgin olive oil

3 tablespoons water, divided

2 tablespoons whole-wheat flour

5 or 6 boneless, skinless chicken breasts

1 large white onion, diced

1 green bell pepper, cored and diced

1 red bell pepper, cored and diced

12 ounces cremini mushrooms, stemmed and chopped

1 (28-ounce) can crushed or diced tomatoes

3½ cups Savory Chicken Broth (page 144) or store-bought chicken broth

4 teaspoons minced garlic

2 tablespoons Italian seasoning

2 tablespoons red-wine vinegar

10 to 12 ounces thin spaghetti

3 (6-ounce) cans tomato paste

Sea salt

Ground black pepper

Fresh thyme leaves, for topping

1 to 1¼ cups grated Parmesan cheese, for topping

1. Coat the bottom of a 6-quart slow cooker with the olive oil.

2. Add 1 tablespoon of the water and whisk in the flour.

3. Add the chicken, onion, green bell pepper, red bell pepper, mushrooms, tomatoes, broth, garlic, Italian seasoning, vinegar, and the remaining 2 tablespoons of water. Mix well. Cover and cook on low for 6 hours, until the chicken has cooked through and the vegetables are soft.

4. Remove the lid and add the spaghetti and tomato paste. Stir gently. Replace the lid and cook for an additional 20 to 30 minutes, until the spaghetti is soft.

5. Turn off the slow cooker. Top with thyme and 2 tablespoons of cheese per serving. Add salt and pepper to taste and serve the chicken warm.

CONTINUED →

Chicken Cacciatore CONTINUED

6. Refrigerate leftovers for up to 1 week, or freeze for up to 2 months.

SERVING RECOMMENDATIONS

Soft Foods: ½ cup
General Foods: 1 cup

Per serving: Calories: 397; Protein: 34g; Fat: 9g; Carbohydrates: 49g; Fiber: 9g; Sugar: 13g; Sodium: 227mg

Indian-Inspired Chicken and Rice

Prep time: 15 minutes
Cook time: 6 hours on low
SERVES 8 TO 10

Made famous in Delhi, the capital region of India, in the 1950s, this now internationally popular warming dish has all the spicy heat I love about Indian cuisine. However, it can also be made with a milder spice profile and is easy to modify to your preferences. It is perfect for your soft-foods stage. Serve it with naan or roti bread.

1 tablespoon extra-virgin olive oil

3 to 3½ pounds boneless, skinless chicken thighs, cut into bite-size pieces

1 large white onion, diced

1 tablespoon minced garlic

1½ tablespoons grated fresh ginger

1 tablespoon curry powder

1 tablespoon garam masala

2 teaspoons ground cumin

1 teaspoon cayenne pepper

1 teaspoon sea salt

½ teaspoon ground black pepper

1 teaspoon coconut sugar

2¼ cups coconut milk

1 (6-ounce) can tomato paste

2 to 2½ cups cooked wild or basmati rice

Plain Greek yogurt, for topping

Freshly squeezed lime juice, for topping

1. Coat the bottom of a 6-quart slow cooker with the olive oil.

2. Add the chicken, onion, garlic, ginger, curry powder, garam masala, cumin, cayenne, salt, black pepper, sugar, coconut milk, and tomato paste. Mix well. Cover and cook on low for 6 hours, until the chicken has cooked through.

3. Turn off the slow cooker. Serve the chicken over ¼ cup of rice per serving. Top with a dollop of Greek yogurt and a squeeze of lime juice.

4. Refrigerate leftovers for up to 5 days, or freeze for up to 1 month.

SERVING RECOMMENDATIONS

Soft Foods: ½ cup
General Foods: 1 cup

Per serving: Calories: 441; Protein: 37g; Fat: 23g; Carbohydrates: 23g; Fiber: 2g; Sugar: 4g; Sodium: 330mg

Lemon Chicken and Broccoli

Prep time: 15 minutes
Cook time: 8 hours 15 minutes on low
SERVES 8 TO 10

This tangy chicken dish is great as a complete meal on its own, providing healing protein and important minerals. Additionally, lemon can support digestion and boost iron absorption. Serve by itself or with ¼ cup of cooked wild rice on the side.

6 teaspoons grated lemon zest, divided

1½ tablespoons Dijon mustard

1 to 2 tablespoons extra-virgin olive oil

2 teaspoons dried oregano

¼ teaspoon salt

½ teaspoon dried thyme

2 pounds bone-in, skin-on chicken thighs

⅓ cup freshly squeezed lemon juice (2 or 3 lemons)

1½ cups Savory Chicken Broth (page 144) or store-bought chicken broth

1 tablespoon butter

2 tablespoons whole-wheat flour or all-purpose gluten-free flour

1 to 2 cups fresh broccoli

1. To make the rub, in a small bowl, combine 2 teaspoons of lemon zest, the mustard, olive oil, oregano, salt, and thyme. Using your fingers or a brush, cover the chicken with the rub.

2. In a 6-quart slow cooker, combine the remaining 4 teaspoons of lemon zest, the lemon juice, broth, butter, and flour. Whisk for 2 minutes.

3. Add the chicken. Cover and cook on low for 8 hours, until the chicken has cooked through and the lemon sauce has thickened.

4. Remove the lid and add the broccoli. Replace the lid and cook for an additional 10 to 15 minutes, until the broccoli is tender.

5. Turn off the slow cooker. Serve the chicken and broccoli warm. Refrigerate leftovers for up to 5 days, or freeze for up to 1 month.

SERVING RECOMMENDATIONS

General Foods: 1 cup

Per serving: Calories: 284; Protein: 20g; Fat: 21g; Carbohydrates: 4g; Fiber: 1g; Sugar: 1g; Sodium: 171mg

Rotisserie-Style Whole Chicken

Prep time: 15 minutes
Cook time: 8 hours on low, plus 5 minutes to rest
SERVES 8 TO 10

This go-with-anything recipe is perfect for when you want to make a large amount of protein ahead. It combines well with just about any rice or vegetable side, and it reheats easily in the microwave or the oven. It's also a protein- and iron-rich option that is safe if you are avoiding major allergens.

1 tablespoon sea salt

1 teaspoon ground black pepper

2 teaspoons smoked paprika

½ teaspoon ground white pepper

½ teaspoon cayenne pepper

½ teaspoon garlic powder

½ teaspoon onion powder

½ teaspoon dried thyme

1 (5- to 6-pound) fresh whole chicken

1. To make the spice rub, in a small bowl, combine the salt, black pepper, paprika, white pepper, cayenne, garlic powder, onion powder, and thyme.

2. Remove the giblets from inside the chicken, and use a paper towel to dry the interior.

3. Place 4 balls of aluminum foil in the bottom of a 6-quart slow cooker (this will be your chicken "rack").

4. Rub the outside and inside of the chicken with the spice rub, coating it well.

5. Place the chicken on the foil balls inside the slow cooker. Cover and cook on low for 8 hours, until the chicken is golden brown and cooked through or a meat thermometer inserted into the thigh or breast reads 165°F.

6. Turn off the slow cooker. Transfer the chicken to a rack or cutting board. Let rest for 5 minutes.

7. Slice the chicken and serve warm.

8. Refrigerate leftovers for up to 1 week, or freeze for up to 2 months.

CONTINUED →

MAKE IT A MEAL

Pair this with ¼ cup of any vegetable or ¼ cup of rice.

TIP

Make a larger batch of the spice rub ahead, and save it for later to speed up prep time.

SERVING RECOMMENDATIONS

Soft Foods: ½ cup
General Foods: 1 cup

Per serving: Calories: 375; Protein: 32g; Fat: 26g; Carbohydrates: 1g; Fiber: 0g; Sugar: 0g; Sodium: 557mg

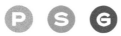

Simple Ground Turkey and Vegetables

Prep time: 15 minutes
Cook time: 3 minutes on high and 7 to 8 hours on low
SERVES 6 TO 8

This versatile recipe can be used for several different meals throughout the week, giving you a protein-, iron-, and fiber-rich dish that you can mix and match with various sides. The ground turkey is a perfect protein addition to your soft-foods menu during your recovery.

3 tablespoons extra-virgin olive oil

1 tablespoon minced garlic

1 large white onion, chopped

3 pounds ground turkey

1 large red bell pepper, cored and chopped

1 large yellow bell pepper, cored and chopped

1 large orange bell pepper, cored and chopped

1 large sweet potato, peeled and chopped

1 large zucchini, peeled and chopped

1 to 1½ cups water

2 teaspoons sea salt

½ teaspoon ground black pepper

3 tablespoons low-sodium soy sauce or coconut aminos

1 tablespoon dried oregano

2 teaspoons paprika

2 teaspoons chopped fresh parsley

½ lemon

1. In a 6-quart slow cooker, combine the olive oil, garlic, and onion. Cook on high, stirring occasionally, for 2 to 3 minutes, until fragrant.

2. Stir in the turkey, red bell pepper, yellow bell pepper, orange bell pepper, sweet potato, and zucchini.

3. Add the water, salt, black pepper, soy sauce, oregano, paprika, parsley, and a squeeze of lemon juice. Mix well. Cover, reduce the heat to low, and cook for 7 to 8 hours, until the turkey has cooked through and the vegetables are soft.

4. Turn off the slow cooker. Serve the turkey and vegetables warm.

5. Refrigerate leftovers for up to 1 week, or freeze for up to 2 months.

MAKE IT A MEAL

For the soft- and general-foods stages, pair this with ¼ cup of any rice or potato side, or use ¼ cup of the leftovers as a filling for tacos, in a hot sandwich on a whole-grain bun, or mixed with rice in a power bowl.

CONTINUED →

Simple Ground Turkey and Vegetables CONTINUED

TIP

To make this recipe for your puree recovery stage, simply use an immersion blender to puree after cooking.

SERVING RECOMMENDATIONS

Pureed Foods: ¼–½ cup
Soft Foods: ½ cup
General Foods: 1 cup

Per serving: Calories: 469; Protein: 48g; Fat: 25g; Carbohydrates: 16g; Fiber: 3g; Sugar: 5g; Sodium: 795mg

Tasty Turkey Meatballs

Prep time: 15 minutes
Cook time: 6 to 7 hours on low
SERVES 6 TO 8

Meatballs made in the slow cooker are tender, savory, and full of flavor—not to mention, super easy! Mix them up, form them, and throw them in. That's it! Full of lean protein, iron, and B vitamins (and fiber from the oats!), they also will provide you with the nutrients you need most during your soft-foods stage of recovery.

1 tablespoon extra-virgin olive oil

1 pound lean ground turkey

1 pound sweet Italian turkey sausage

¾ cup rolled oats

¼ cup fresh grated Parmesan cheese, plus more for topping (optional)

3 large eggs

¼ cup finely chopped fresh parsley, plus more for topping (optional)

¼ cup dried basil

½ teaspoon sea salt

½ teaspoon ground black pepper

2 teaspoons minced garlic

1 (28-ounce) jar no-sugar-added marinara sauce

1 (15-ounce) can crushed tomatoes

1 (15-ounce) can tomato sauce

1½ to 2 cups cooked whole-wheat pasta

1. Coat the bottom of a 6-quart slow cooker with the olive oil.

2. In a large bowl, combine the ground turkey, turkey sausage, oats, cheese, eggs, parsley, basil, salt, black pepper, and garlic. Stir.

3. Form the turkey mixture into 1½-inch balls. Arrange the balls in a single layer on the bottom of the slow cooker until the bottom is covered (you will probably have some meatballs left).

4. In a separate large bowl, mix together the marinara sauce, crushed tomatoes, and tomato sauce.

5. Pour one-third to half of the tomato mixture over top of the meatballs.

6. Repeat another layer of meatballs, and cover with the remaining sauce. Cover and cook on low for 6 to 7 hours, until the meatballs have cooked through.

CONTINUED →

7. Turn off the slow cooker. Top with additional parsley and cheese (if using).

8. Serve the meatballs warm over ¼ cup of pasta per serving. Refrigerate leftovers for up to 1 week, or freeze for up to 3 months.

TIP

Use 85 percent lean ground beef if you prefer.

SERVING RECOMMENDATIONS

Soft Foods: ½ cup
General Foods: 1 cup

Per serving: Calories: 469; Protein: 39g; Fat: 20g; Carbohydrates: 37g; Fiber: 8g; Sugar: 10g; Sodium: 848mg

Turkey-Stuffed Peppers

Prep time: 15 minutes
Cook time: 7 hours 45 minutes on low
SERVES 6

I love stuffed peppers because they are an easy meal that provides you with protein, starch, and vegetables in one dish! They are also versatile with cheese and sauce, so you can create the flavor you want. These are perfect for your soft-foods and general-foods stages of recovery. You'll meet your protein and fiber needs in one shot.

1 pound lean ground turkey

1 tablespoon extra-virgin olive oil

2 teaspoons minced garlic

1 medium white onion, diced

1½ cups cooked rice

1½ teaspoons sea salt

¼ teaspoon ground black pepper

1 tablespoon dried basil

1 tablespoon dried parsley

6 yellow, orange, or red bell peppers, tops cut off and reserved, cored

¼ cup water

1 (24-ounce) jar marinara sauce

2 cups shredded mozzarella cheese

Grated Parmesan cheese, for topping

Fresh parsley, for topping

1. In a large bowl, combine the turkey, olive oil, garlic, onion, rice, salt, black pepper, basil, and dried parsley. Mix well.

2. Stuff each bell pepper evenly with the turkey mixture, then cover each bell pepper with its top.

3. Pour the water into a 6-quart slow cooker, then place each bell pepper inside. Cover and cook on low for 7 hours, until the turkey has cooked through.

4. Remove the lid, pour the marinara sauce over the peppers, and sprinkle the mozzarella cheese evenly over the top of the sauce and bell peppers. Replace the lid, and cook for an additional 30 to 45 minutes, until the cheese has melted.

5. Turn off the slow cooker. Top with Parmesan cheese and fresh parsley. Serve the peppers warm.

6. Refrigerate leftovers for up to 5 days, or freeze for up to 1 month.

CONTINUED →

Turkey-Stuffed Peppers CONTINUED

TIP

For a different flavor, swap out the marinara for pesto in the same amount. You can also use Parmesan instead of mozzarella (follow the same cooking instructions). Use 85 percent lean ground beef, ground pork, or ground chicken if you prefer.

SERVING RECOMMENDATIONS

Soft Foods: ½ cup
General Foods: 1 cup

Per serving: Calories: 393; Protein: 28g; Fat: 17g; Carbohydrates: 34g; Fiber: 4g; Sugar: 5g; Sodium: 587mg

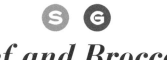

Beef and Broccoli

Prep time: 15 minutes
Cook time: 6 hours 30 minutes on low
SERVES 6

This dish originates from the Chinese dish *Gai Lan Chao Niu Rou* ("Chinese Broccoli Fried Beef"). Chinese broccoli, gai lan, is a large, leafy green vegetable with a bulky stem. Early immigrants to the United States couldn't find this vegetable, so American broccoli was used instead. Protein- and fiber-rich, this dish is perfect for your soft-foods stage!

2 pounds boneless beef chuck roast, thinly sliced

1 cup beef broth

1 tablespoon extra-virgin olive oil

½ cup low-sodium soy sauce or coconut aminos

¼ cup coconut sugar

2 teaspoons minced garlic

¼ cup cornstarch

1 (14-ounce) bag frozen broccoli

1½ cups cooked rice

1. Place the beef in a 6-quart slow cooker.

2. In a medium bowl, whisk together the broth, olive oil, soy sauce, sugar, and garlic.

3. Pour the mixture over the beef in the slow cooker. Mix well so the beef is coated thoroughly. Cover and cook on low for 5 to 6 hours, until the beef has cooked through.

4. Remove the lid and transfer ¼ cup of the liquid to a small bowl.

5. Add the cornstarch to the bowl, and whisk to combine. Then, mix the slurry back into the ingredients in the slow cooker.

6. Add the broccoli and mix well. Replace the lid and cook for an additional 30 minutes.

7. Turn off the slow cooker. Serve the beef and broccoli warm over ¼ cup of rice per serving.

8. Refrigerate leftovers for up to 5 days, or freeze for up to 2 months.

SERVING RECOMMENDATIONS

Soft Foods: ½ cup
General Foods: 1 cup

Per serving: Calories: 450; Protein: 34g; Fat: 21g; Carbohydrates: 32g; Fiber: 2g; Sugar: 9g; Sodium: 893mg

Beef Bourguignon

Prep time: 15 minutes
Cook time: 5 minutes on high and 6 to 7 hours on low
SERVES 6 TO 8

Chef Auguste Escoffier is credited with being the first to publish a recipe for this dish in France around 1903, and it quickly evolved from a simple, affordable dish to a trendy French entrée. The texture makes it a perfect soft-foods dish for your recovery, and it also provides essential protein, iron, B vitamins, fiber, and beta-carotene (vitamin A).

2 tablespoons extra-virgin olive oil

2 teaspoons minced garlic

1 medium yellow onion, chopped

6 bacon slices, diced

3 cups red wine

1 cup beef broth

3 tablespoons tomato paste

½ teaspoon dried thyme

1½ cups sliced carrots

1 pound cremini mushrooms, halved

2 tablespoons dried parsley

1 or 2 bay leaves

3 pounds beef chuck roast, cut into 1- to 2-inch pieces

1 teaspoon sea salt

1 teaspoon ground black pepper

1 tablespoon cornstarch

1 tablespoon water

1. In a 6-quart slow cooker, combine the olive oil, garlic, onion, and bacon. Cook on high, stirring every minute or so, for 4 to 5 minutes, until fragrant.

2. Meanwhile, in a large bowl, combine the wine, broth, and tomato paste. Mix well.

3. Stir the thyme, carrots, mushrooms, parsley, and bay leaf into the wine mixture.

4. Pat the beef dry. Season with the salt and black pepper and add to the slow cooker.

5. Pour the wine mixture over the beef and stir to combine.

6. Add the cornstarch and water. Stir. Cover, reduce the heat to low, and cook for 6 to 7 hours, until the beef is tender and cooked through.

7. Turn off the slow cooker. Discard the bay leaf. Serve the stew warm.

8. Refrigerate leftovers for up to 1 week, or freeze for up to 2 months.

MAKE IT A MEAL

Serve with ¼ cup of baked potato, ¼ cup of mashed potatoes, a slice of whole-grain bread, or ¼ cup of cooked whole-grain spaghetti.

SERVING RECOMMENDATIONS

Soft Foods: ½ cup
General Foods: 1 cup

Per serving: Calories: 731; Protein: 50g; Fat: 44g; Carbohydrates: 14g; Fiber: 2g; Sugar: 6g; Sodium: 591mg

Classic Pot Roast with Vegetables

Prep time: 15 minutes
Cook time: 4 minutes on high and 9 to 10 hours on low
SERVES 8

A classic comfort dish, this entrée will deliver on savory flavor, tender texture, and nutrition. Perfect for your soft-foods phase, find your protein, fiber, and vegetables all in one dish here. It's also rich in B vitamins, iron, and vitamin A.

2 tablespoons extra-virgin olive oil

4 medium potatoes, peeled and diced

5 large carrots, sliced

1 medium yellow onion, diced

1 teaspoon minced garlic

4 pounds beef chuck roast

1 teaspoon sea salt

1 teaspoon ground black pepper

2½ cups beef broth

1½ tablespoons Worcestershire sauce

1 teaspoon dried basil

3 tablespoons cornstarch

Chopped fresh parsley, for topping

1. In a 6-quart slow cooker, combine the olive oil, potatoes, carrots, onion, and garlic. Cook on high, stirring occasionally, for 3 to 4 minutes, until the vegetables begin to sizzle.

2. Meanwhile, season the beef with the salt and black pepper. Place on top of the vegetables in the slow cooker.

3. In a medium bowl, combine the broth, Worcestershire sauce, and basil. Mix well.

4. Pour the mixture into the slow cooker. Cover, reduce the heat to low, and cook for 9 to 10 hours, until the beef is easily shredded and the vegetables are very soft.

5. Remove the lid and transfer ½ cup of the liquid from the slow cooker to a bowl.

6. Whisk the cornstarch into the bowl until the mixture has thickened. Then, mix the slurry back into the ingredients in the slow cooker, making sure it is well combined with the vegetables and remaining liquid. Replace the lid and cook for an additional 2 to 3 minutes, until the gravy has thickened.

7. Turn off the slow cooker. Transfer the beef and vegetables to a serving platter.

8. Pour the gravy over the beef and garnish with parsley. Serve warm.

9. Refrigerate leftovers for up to 1 week, or freeze for up to 2 months.

TIP

If you have the time and energy, you can pan-sear the roast in a separate pan in olive oil over medium-high heat for 4 to 5 minutes before putting it in the slow cooker. This creates a lovely, flavorful crust on the outside of the roast.

SERVING RECOMMENDATIONS

Soft Foods: ½ cup
General Foods: 1 cup

Per serving: Calories: 575; Protein: 46g; Fat: 31g; Carbohydrates: 28g; Fiber: 4g; Sugar: 4g; Sodium: 390mg

(S) (G)

Easy Pork Tenderloin

Prep time: 10 minutes
Cook time: 3 minutes on high and 6 hours on low
SERVES 8

Pork tenderloin can go with anything, which is what makes this recipe a great weeknight go-to. Its versatility means you can make it once for the week and then switch up the sides, as desired, for variety. Perfect for your soft-foods stage, pork also provides essential protein, B vitamins, iron, zinc, and selenium.

2 tablespoons extra-virgin olive oil

1 medium yellow onion, diced

1 teaspoon garlic powder

1 teaspoon onion powder

1 teaspoon sea salt

1 teaspoon ground black pepper

¼ cup coconut sugar

1 tablespoon chili powder

1 tablespoon smoked paprika

4 pounds boneless pork loin

2 cups Savory Chicken Broth (page 144) or store-bought chicken broth

1. In a 6-quart slow cooker, combine the olive oil and onion. Cook on high, stirring occasionally, for 2 to 3 minutes, until the onion begins to sizzle.

2. In a small bowl, mix together the garlic powder, onion powder, salt, black pepper, sugar, chili powder, and paprika.

3. Thoroughly season the pork with the spice mixture. Add to the slow cooker.

4. Add the broth. Cover, reduce the heat to low, and cook for 6 hours, until the pork has cooked through.

5. Turn off the slow cooker. Spoon the broth from the bottom of the slow cooker over the meat, and serve warm.

6. Refrigerate leftovers for up to 1 week, or freeze for up to 3 months.

SERVING RECOMMENDATIONS

Soft Foods: ½ cup
General Foods: 1 cup

Per serving: Calories: 445; Protein: 49g; Fat: 22g; Carbohydrates: 9g; Fiber: 1g; Sugar: 7g; Sodium: 282mg

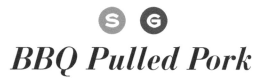

BBQ Pulled Pork

Prep time: 10 minutes
Cook time: 8 hours on low
SERVES 8

This pulled pork will hit your sweet, savory, and spicy taste buds all at once! It's a great option when starting out in your soft-foods stage, given the pork texture and moisture content. You'll also achieve your protein, iron, and B vitamin goals. Add more fiber with a baked potato or vegetable side.

4 pounds pork roast

1 teaspoon sea salt

1 teaspoon ground black pepper

1 tablespoon garlic powder

1 tablespoon chili powder

1 (32-ounce) bottle barbecue sauce

½ cup apple cider vinegar

½ cup Savory Chicken Broth (page 144) or store-bought chicken broth

1 tablespoon Worcestershire sauce

¼ cup coconut sugar

4 whole-grain buns, halved

1. Season the pork thoroughly with the salt, black pepper, garlic powder, and chili powder. Place the pork in a 6-quart slow cooker.

2. Add the barbecue sauce, vinegar, broth, Worcestershire sauce, and sugar. Cover and cook on low for 8 hours, until the pork has cooked through and can be shredded easily.

3. Remove the lid and transfer the pork to a cutting board or platter. Shred it using 2 forks, then return it to the slow cooker. Mix well to coat with the sauce.

4. Turn off the slow cooker. Serve the pork warm on the buns. Refrigerate leftovers for up to 1 week, or freeze for up to 3 months.

TIP

Once you reach the general-foods stage, serve with coleslaw on the side.

SERVING RECOMMENDATIONS

Soft Foods: ½ cup
General Foods: 1 cup

Per serving: Calories: 666; Protein: 51g; Fat: 21g; Carbohydrates: 65g; Fiber: 3g; Sugar: 46g; Sodium: 1,042mg

Creole Chicken and Sausage

Prep time: 10 minutes
Cook time: 7 hours 30 minutes on low
SERVES 8

Creole culture flourished in 18th-century Louisiana before the territory was sold to the United States in 1803. Dishes are marked by the abundant use of local fresh seafood, fresh tomatoes, cayenne, and rich sauces—a few of which you'll see in this dish that's great for the soft-foods phase!

1½ pounds boneless, skinless chicken breasts

2½ cups thinly sliced andouille sausage

1 medium yellow onion, diced

2 teaspoons minced garlic

1½ cups Savory Chicken Broth (page 144) or store-bought chicken broth

1 (14½-ounce) can diced tomatoes, drained

1/4 cup tomato paste

½ cup tomato sauce

1 tablespoon Creole seasoning

¼ cup cayenne pepper

1 tablespoon coconut sugar

1 (15-ounce) can black or kidney beans, drained and rinsed

Sliced scallions, green parts only, for topping

2 cups cooked brown or wild rice

1. In a 6-quart slow cooker, combine the chicken, sausage, onion, garlic, broth, diced tomatoes, tomato paste, tomato sauce, Creole seasoning, cayenne, and sugar. Cover and cook on low for 6 to 7 hours, until the chicken and sausage have cooked through and the vegetables are soft.

2. Remove the lid and transfer the chicken to a cutting board or platter. Shred it using 2 forks, then return it to the slow cooker. Mix well.

3. Stir in the beans. Replace the lid and cook for an additional 20 to 30 minutes, until the beans are heated and easily mashed.

4. Turn off the slow cooker. Garnish with scallions (do not add if you are at the soft-foods stage), and serve the chicken and sausage warm over ¼ cup of rice per serving. Refrigerate leftovers for up to 1 week, or freeze for up to 2 months.

SERVING RECOMMENDATIONS

Soft Foods: ½ cup   **General Foods:** 1 cup

Per serving: Calories: 316; Protein: 28g; Fat: 10g; Carbohydrates: 29g; Fiber: 6g; Sugar: 6g; Sodium: 358mg

Sausage and Peppers over Rice

Prep time: 15 minutes
Cook time: 6 to 7 hours on low
SERVES 8 TO 10

Fill up on protein, fiber, antioxidants, and vegetables with this slow cooker version of a classic favorite. Choosing rice or potatoes over a hoagie may be easier on your digestion during the soft-foods stage while also boosting your fiber intake. Adding cheese at the end also provides a protein and calcium boost.

2 tablespoons extra-virgin olive oil

2 pounds sweet Italian sausage links

2 red bell peppers, cored and sliced

1 orange or yellow bell pepper, cored and sliced

1 medium yellow onion, cut into strips

1 (15-ounce) jar red pasta sauce

2 teaspoons minced garlic

1 teaspoon Italian seasoning

1 teaspoon sea salt

¼ teaspoon red pepper flakes or cayenne pepper

1 to 2 cups shredded mozzarella cheese

2 to 2½ cups cooked brown or wild rice

1. Coat the bottom of a 6-quart slow cooker with the olive oil. Heat on low for 2 to 3 minutes.

2. Add the sausage, red bell peppers, orange bell pepper, onion, pasta sauce, garlic, Italian seasoning, salt, and red pepper flakes. Mix well. Cover and cook for 6 to 7 hours, until the sausage has cooked through and the vegetables are soft.

3. Turn off the slow cooker. Remove the lid and sprinkle with the cheese.

4. Serve the sausage and peppers warm over ¼ cup of rice per serving. Refrigerate leftovers for up to 1 week, or freeze for up to 2 months.

TIP

You can also serve this dish with cauliflower rice, ½ of a whole-grain hoagie, or ¼ cup of baked potato instead of brown or wild rice.

SERVING RECOMMENDATIONS

Soft Foods: ½ cup
General Foods: 1 cup

Per serving: Calories: 318; Protein: 24g; Fat: 17g; Carbohydrates: 19g; Fiber: 3g; Sugar: 4g; Sodium: 967mg

Maple-Balsamic Lamb Shoulder

Prep time: 15 minutes
Cook time: 8 hours 10 minutes on low
SERVES 6 TO 8

Rich in tangy, sweet flavor, this dish may have you wanting seconds! The lamb becomes quite tender in the slow cooker, and the balsamic vinegar helps facilitate this. Rich in protein, B vitamins, and iron, you will be meeting your essential nutrition goals here. And a baked potato or vegetable side brings fiber to the game.

2 tablespoons extra-virgin olive oil

3 to 4 pounds lamb shoulder, trimmed of excess fat

1 cup beef broth or chicken broth

1 cup aged balsamic vinegar

1 tablespoon onion powder

⅔ cup pure maple syrup

1 teaspoon minced garlic

1 tablespoon dried oregano

2 teaspoons dried sage

1 teaspoon sea salt

1 teaspoon ground black pepper

2 tablespoons feta cheese, for topping

Arugula, for topping

1. Coat the bottom of a 6-quart slow cooker with the olive oil. Heat on low for 2 to 3 minutes.

2. Place the lamb in the slow cooker, with the fattiest part on top.

3. Add the broth, vinegar, onion powder, maple syrup, garlic, oregano, sage, salt, and black pepper on top of the lamb, letting the liquid fall over the sides of the lamb. Cover and cook on low for 7 to 8 hours, until the lamb is tender and cooked through.

4. Remove the lid and transfer the lamb to a cutting board or platter. Cut it into 1- to 2-inch chunks, or shred it using 2 forks. Return it to the slow cooker and stir. Replace the lid and cook for an additional 5 to 10 minutes.

5. Turn off the slow cooker. Top with the cheese and arugula. (Depending on how you feel, you may want to save arugula for later in the soft-foods stage or for the general-foods stage.) Serve the lamb warm.

6. Refrigerate leftovers for up to 1 week, or freeze for up to 2 months.

You can serve this with cauliflower rice, ½ of a whole-grain sandwich bun, or ¼ cup of cooked brown or wild rice.

Soft Foods: ½ cup
General Foods: 1 cup

Per serving: Calories: 765; Protein: 39g; Fat: 52g; Carbohydrates: 32g; Fiber: 1g; Sugar: 28g; Sodium: 345mg

Moroccan-Inspired Lamb Shanks

Prep time: 15 minutes
Cook time: 10 minutes on high and 5 to 6 hours on low
SERVES 6 TO 8

Moroccan cuisine is known for its use of a variety of spices, including cumin, paprika, ginger, cinnamon, coriander, and turmeric, as well as apricots, dates, and legumes. In this dish, the combination of flavorful spices with sweet apricots and hearty chickpeas creates a burst of flavor and texture while still being gentle on your healing stomach.

2 tablespoons extra-virgin olive oil

1 large white onion, diced

1 teaspoon minced garlic

1 tablespoon ground cumin

2 teaspoons ground coriander

1 teaspoon ground turmeric

1 teaspoon paprika

1 tablespoon minced fresh ginger

½ teaspoon ground cinnamon

1 teaspoon sea salt

1 teaspoon ground black pepper

6 or 7 lamb shanks, trimmed of excess fat

4 cups Savory Chicken Broth (page 144) or store-bought chicken broth

1 large sweet potato, peeled and chopped

1 (15-ounce) can chickpeas, drained and rinsed

1 cup dried apricots

2 medium tomatoes, peeled and chopped

¾ to 1 cup feta cheese, for topping (optional)

Arugula, for topping (optional)

1. Coat the bottom of a 6-quart slow cooker with the olive oil.

2. Set the heat to high. Add the onion and cook for 2 to 3 minutes, until fragrant.

3. Meanwhile, in a small bowl, combine the garlic, cumin, coriander, turmeric, paprika, ginger, cinnamon, salt, and black pepper.

4. Thoroughly coat each lamb shank with the spice mixture, and add them to the slow cooker. Sear for 2 to 3 minutes per side.

5. Add the broth, remaining spice mixture (if any), the sweet potato, chickpeas, apricots, and tomatoes. Mix well. Cover, reduce the heat to low, and cook for 5 to 6 hours, until the lamb shanks have cooked through.

6. Turn off the slow cooker. Top with 2 tablespoons of cheese per serving (if using) and arugula (if using). (Depending on how you feel, you may want to save arugula for later in the soft-foods stage or for the general-foods stage.) Serve the lamb warm.

7. Refrigerate leftovers for up to 5 days, or freeze for up to 2 months.

TIP

You can serve this with ¼ cup of cauliflower rice or brown or wild rice for a gluten-free option.

SERVING RECOMMENDATIONS

Soft Foods: ½ cup
General Foods: 1 cup

Per serving: Calories: 414; Protein: 29g; Fat: 19g; Carbohydrates: 35g; Fiber: 7g; Sugar: 17g; Sodium: 304mg

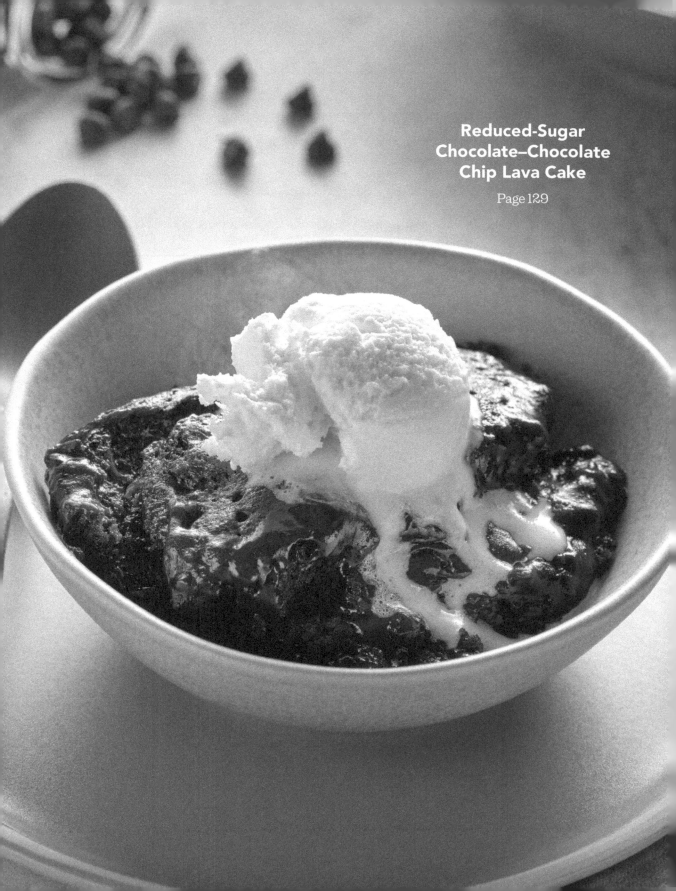

Reduced-Sugar Chocolate–Chocolate Chip Lava Cake

Page 129

7

Desserts

Ⓛ LIQUIDS   Ⓢ SOFT FOODS   PUREED FOODS   Ⓖ GENERAL FOODS FOR LIFE

(P) (S) (G)
Cran-Apple Pear Compote

Prep time: 10 minutes
Cook time: 6 to 8 hours on low
SERVES 4 TO 6

Dive into the rich flavor of fall with this sweet, low-sugar dessert. Apples and pears provide essential fiber for smooth digestion and satiety, while cranberries add natural sweetness and texture. Rich in phytonutrients and antioxidants, this dessert will satisfy your sweet tooth and fight inflammation. Serve warm for the richest flavor.

¾ cup no-sugar-added cranberry juice

¼ cup pure maple syrup

2 medium apples, peeled, cored, and chopped

2 medium pears, peeled, cored, and chopped

⅓ cup dried cranberries

1 to 1½ cups no-sugar-added vanilla ice cream (optional)

1. In a 6-quart slow cooker, combine the cranberry juice, maple syrup, apples, pears, and dried cranberries. Cover and cook on low for 6 to 8 hours, until the apples and pears are soft and easily mashed.

2. Turn off the slow cooker. Serve the compote warm on its own or with ¼ cup of ice cream per serving.

3. Refrigerate leftovers for up to 5 days, or freeze for up to 1 month.

TIP

Set the cook time for 8 hours (rather than 6) for a softer texture. To make this recipe for your puree recovery stage, simply use an immersion blender to puree after cooking.

SERVING RECOMMENDATIONS

Pureed Foods: ¼–½ cup
Soft Foods: ½ cup
General Foods: 1 cup

Per serving: Calories: 206; Protein: 1g; Fat: 0g; Carbohydrates: 54g; Fiber: 6g; Sugar: 42g; Sodium: 5mg

Reduced-Sugar Chocolate–Chocolate Chip Lava Cake

Prep time: 15 minutes
Cook time: 4 to 5 hours on low
SERVES 10 TO 12

Recovering from bariatric surgery doesn't mean you can't enjoy a little chocolate! This lava cake will satisfy chocolate cravings and help you manage your sugar intake. It is made with sugar-free cake and pudding mixes; coconut sugar, which causes a smaller blood-glucose spike; and semisweet chocolate chips, which help keep added sugar consumption to a minimum. It's also a perfect dessert choice for your soft-foods stage of recovery.

1 tablespoon coconut oil, plus ½ cup

1 (16-ounce) box sugar-free devil's food cake mix, such as Pillsbury

1¼ cups 2 percent milk, plus 2 cups

3 large eggs

1 (4-ounce) box sugar-free instant chocolate pudding mix, such as Jell-O or Royal brands

¾ cup coconut sugar

1 (12-ounce) bag semisweet chocolate chips

2½ to 3 cups no-sugar-added vanilla ice cream (optional)

1¼ to 1½ cups light whipped cream, for topping (optional)

1. Coat the bottom and sides of a 6-quart slow cooker with 1 tablespoon of coconut oil.

2. To make the cake batter, in a large bowl, beat together the cake mix, 1¼ cups of milk, the remaining ½ cup of coconut oil, and the eggs until thoroughly combined.

3. Pour the cake batter into the slow cooker in an even layer.

4. To make the topping, in a medium bowl, combine the pudding mix, sugar, and 2 cups of milk.

5. Pour the topping over the cake batter. Do not stir.

6. Sprinkle the chocolate chips over the topping. Cover and cook on low for 4 to 5 hours, until the top is spongy and the inside is gooey.

7. Turn off the slow cooker. Serve the cake warm with ¼ cup of ice cream per serving (if using) or 2 tablespoons of light whipped cream per serving (if using).

8. Refrigerate leftovers for up to 5 days, or freeze for up to 2 months.

CONTINUED →

Reduced-Sugar Chocolate–Chocolate Chip Lava Cake CONTINUED

TIP

Make this completely sugar-free by using Splenda or stevia instead of coconut sugar and by using sugar-free chocolate chips.

Serve with ¼ cup of plain Greek yogurt per serving instead of ice cream for more protein.

SERVING RECOMMENDATIONS

Soft Foods: ½ cup
General Foods: 1 cup

Per serving: Calories: 584; Protein: 9g; Fat: 30g; Carbohydrates: 76g; Fiber: 4g; Sugar: 32g; Sodium: 632mg

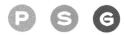

Easy Crustless Pumpkin Pie

Prep time: 15 minutes
Cook time: 3 to 4 hours on low, plus 30 minutes to cool and 3 hours to chill
SERVES 8 TO 10

This simple, easy version of pumpkin pie is a perfect soft-foods dessert for your recovery. Being lower in sugar, you can eat your pumpkin pie without feeling like you're overdoing it. Cornstarch and pumpkin puree also add a little fiber for further blood-sugar management and satiety.

1 tablespoon coconut oil

¾ cup coconut sugar, plus ½ teaspoon

4 teaspoons cornstarch

¼ teaspoon sea salt

2 teaspoons pumpkin pie spice

½ teaspoon baking powder

1 (15-ounce) can pumpkin puree

1 cup heavy (whipping) cream

2 large eggs, beaten

2 tablespoons butter, melted

2 to 2½ cups no-sugar-added vanilla ice cream (optional)

1 to 1¼ cups light whipped cream, for topping (optional)

1. Coat the bottom and sides of a 6-quart slow cooker with the coconut oil.

2. In a large bowl, combine ¾ cup of sugar, the cornstarch, salt, pumpkin pie spice, and baking powder. Pour into the slow cooker.

3. In a separate large bowl, combine the pumpkin puree, cream, eggs, butter, and remaining ½ teaspoon of sugar. Pour into the slow cooker, and mix gently until the dry and wet ingredients are well combined. Cover and cook on low for 3 to 4 hours, until the middle is set and no longer gooey.

4. Turn off the slow cooker. Remove the stoneware crock (inner cooking vessel) and place on a cooling rack. Remove the lid. Let the pie cool for 20 to 30 minutes, until room temperature. Then, cover and refrigerate for 3 hours.

5. Serve the pie chilled with ¼ cup of vanilla ice cream per serving (if using) or 2 tablespoons of light whipped cream per serving (if using).

6. Refrigerate leftovers for up to 1 week, or freeze for up to 3 months.

CONTINUED →

Easy Crustless Pumpkin Pie CONTINUED

TIP

To make this recipe for your puree recovery stage, cool and chill the pie as directed, then use an immersion blender to puree when ready to enjoy.

SERVING RECOMMENDATIONS

Pureed Foods: ¼–½ cup
Soft Foods: ½ cup
General Foods: 1 cup

Per serving: Calories: 187; Protein: 3g; Fat: 17g; Carbohydrates: 7g; Fiber: 2g; Sugar: 3g; Sodium: 116mg

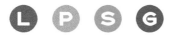

Cinnamon Apples and Pears

Prep time: 10 minutes
Cook time: 4 to 6 hours on low, plus 30 minutes to cool and 3 hours to chill
SERVES 8 TO 10

If you're craving a simple fruit dessert with a slightly spicy twist, this is it! Slow-cooking apples and pears caramelizes them, while the cinnamon adds a kick. Cooked apples and pears are also perfect for your soft-foods recovery stage. You can even puree this after cooking for your liquids phase if desired.

2 (14½-ounce) cans no-sugar-added sliced pears, drained

4 cups sliced peeled apples (3 or 4 medium apples)

1 tablespoon coconut oil

2 teaspoons lemon juice

1 teaspoon ground cinnamon

1 to 2 tablespoons honey (optional)

2 to 2½ cups no-sugar-added vanilla ice cream (optional)

1 to 1¼ cups light whipped cream, for topping (optional)

1. In a large bowl, toss together the pears, apples, and coconut oil. Pour into a 6-quart slow cooker.

2. Add the lemon juice and cinnamon. Stir gently.

3. Gently stir in the honey (if using). Cover and cook on low for 4 to 6 hours, until the pears and apples are soft.

4. Turn off the slow cooker. Remove the stoneware crock (inner cooking vessel) and place on a cooling rack. Remove the lid. Let the dessert cool for 20 to 30 minutes, until room temperature. Then, cover and refrigerate for 2 to 3 hours.

5. Serve the pears and apples chilled with ¼ cup of ice cream per serving (if using) or 2 tablespoons of light whipped cream per serving (if using).

6. Refrigerate leftovers for up to 1 week, or freeze for up to 3 months.

CONTINUED →

Cinnamon Apples and Pears CONTINUED

Per serving: Calories: 107; Protein: 1g; Fat: 2g; Carbohydrates: 23g; Fiber: 4g; Sugar: 16g; Sodium: 1mg

Creamy Vanilla Tapioca Pudding

Prep time: 10 minutes
Cook time: 6 hours on low, plus 30 minutes to cool
and 2 to 3 hours to chill if desired
SERVES 12 TO 14

This creamy and gentle dessert may be particularly calming for an upset stomach during your recovery. Perfect for your soft-foods stage, this pudding provides a little protein while keeping your sugar intake under control. It is great served warm or cold with fruit or chocolate flavors.

5 cups 2 percent milk

2½ cups heavy (whipping) cream

2½ cups water

1½ cups coconut sugar

1 cup small pearl tapioca

4 large eggs, beaten

1 teaspoon vanilla extract

Whipped cream, fresh fruit, cocoa powder, or ground cinnamon, for topping (optional)

1. In a 6-quart slow cooker, combine the milk, cream, water, sugar, tapioca, and eggs.

2. Cover and cook on low for 6 hours, until thick and creamy.

3. Turn off the slow cooker. Stir in the vanilla. If you want to serve the pudding chilled, remove the stoneware crock (inner cooking vessel) and place on a cooling rack. Remove the lid. Let the pudding cool for 20 to 30 minutes. Then, cover and refrigerate for 2 to 3 hours.

4. Serve the pudding warm or chilled with whipped cream, fresh fruit, cocoa powder, or cinnamon (if using).

5. Refrigerate leftovers for up to 1 week, or freeze for up to 3 months.

TIP

Make this vegan by using coconut milk in place of milk, coconut cream in place of heavy cream, and ¼ cup of unsweetened applesauce per chicken egg.

SERVING RECOMMENDATIONS

Soft Foods: ½ cup

General Foods: 1 cup

Per serving: Calories: 393; Protein: 6g; Fat: 22g; Carbohydrates: 43g; Fiber: 0g; Sugar: 32g; Sodium: 91mg

Crème Brûlée with Berries

Prep time: 10 minutes
Cook time: 2 to 2½ hours on low, plus 20 minutes
to cool and 2 to 3 hours to chill
SERVES 4

Crème brûlée may seem fancy and complex, but this recipe will show you how easy it can be. Gentle enough on a healing stomach, this is a great choice for both the liquids (if not adding toppings) and pureed-foods stages of recovery. And the Greek yogurt adds extra protein and calcium for a more nutritious dessert.

1½ cups plain Greek yogurt

½ cup 2 percent milk

1 tablespoon vanilla extract

6 large egg yolks

⅓ cup coconut sugar, plus more for topping

Assorted berries or light whipped cream, for topping (if using)

1. Line the bottom of a 6-quart slow cooker with parchment paper. Place four 3- to 4-inch ramekins in the slow cooker (try to keep them separate from one another).

2. To make the custard mixture, in a medium bowl, combine the yogurt and milk. Mix well.

3. One at a time, whisk in the vanilla, egg yolks, and sugar until well combined.

4. Fill each ramekin three-fourths full of the custard mixture.

5. Drape paper towels along the edge or seal of the slow cooker (around the top, to prevent excessive condensation) before securing the lid. Cook on low for 2 to 2½ hours, until the custard is set and jiggly.

6. Remove the lid. Carefully transfer the ramekins to a cooling rack. Let cool for 10 to 20 minutes, until room temperature. Then, cover with plastic wrap and refrigerate for 2 to 3 hours.

7. If desired, top each serving with a sprinkle of sugar, and using a chef's torch, toast the sugar for a few seconds, until brown and bubbling. Otherwise, serve chilled with berries or whipped cream (if using).

8. Refrigerate leftovers for up to 1 week, or freeze for up to 3 months.

If you are in your liquids or puree recovery phase, serve the custard on its own with no toppings.

If you don't have Greek yogurt, use the same amount of heavy cream instead.

SERVING RECOMMENDATIONS

Liquids: ¼–½ cup
Pureed Foods: ¼–½ cup
Soft Foods: ½ cup
General Foods: 1 cup

Per serving: Calories: 229; Protein: 8g; Fat: 10g; Carbohydrates: 24g; Fiber: 0g; Sugar: 23g; Sodium: 70mg

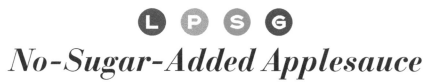

No-Sugar-Added Applesauce

Prep time: 15 minutes
Cook time: 4 hours on low
SERVES 6 TO 8

My favorite way to serve homemade applesauce is warm with a little whipped cream. It tastes and feels decadent while still minimizing your sugar intake and providing fiber. You can use your favorite apples or experiment with different varieties—every combination will have a slightly different flavor. When thoroughly blended, you can enjoy this for your liquids phase, and a slightly chunkier version is great during your soft-foods phase.

Nonstick cooking spray, for coating the slow cooker

2½ pounds green apples, peeled, cored, and sliced (6 or 7 apples)

2½ pounds red apples, peeled, cored and sliced (6 or 7 apples)

Juice of 1 lemon

1 to 2 teaspoons ground cinnamon

⅛ teaspoon ground allspice

Greek yogurt, whipped cream, coconut flakes, or raisins, for topping (optional)

1. Lightly coat the bottom and sides of a 6-quart slow cooker with cooking spray.

2. Add the green apples, red apples, lemon juice, cinnamon, and allspice. Mix well.

3. Cover and cook on low for 4 hours, until the apples are very soft.

4. Turn off the slow cooker. Using an immersion blender, blend the apples to your preferred consistency. If you want a chunkier applesauce, limit the blending time. If you want a smoother texture (like in your liquids and puree recovery phases), thoroughly blend in small batches. (You can also transfer the apples to a regular blender.)

5. Serve the applesauce at room temperature, chilled, or warm with Greek yogurt, whipped cream, coconut flakes, or raisins (if using).

6. Refrigerate leftovers for up to 2 weeks, or freeze for up to 2 months.

If you're in the liquids phase of recovery, serve with no toppings. If you're in the puree phase, limit toppings to only ¼ cup of Greek yogurt.

SERVING RECOMMENDATIONS

Liquids: ¼–½ cup
Pureed Foods: ¼–½ cup
Soft Foods: ½ cup
General Foods: 1 cup

Per serving: Calories: 199; Protein: 1g; Fat: 1g; Carbohydrates: 53g; Fiber: 9g; Sugar: 39g; Sodium: 4mg

L P S G

Better-for-You Hot Chocolate

Prep time: 10 minutes
Cook time: 2 hours on low
SERVES 12

Step up your hot chocolate with this better-for-you slow cooker version! It flips traditional hot chocolate upside down with more protein and less sugar—exactly what you need during your various phases of recovery. Happy sipping!

6 cups 2 percent milk

5 cups whole milk

1 cup heavy (whipping) cream

½ cup coconut sugar

⅓ cup dark chocolate chips

½ cup unsweetened cocoa powder

2 teaspoons vanilla extract

Powdered sugar, sea salt, or cocoa powder, for topping

1. In a 6-quart slow cooker, combine the 2 percent milk, whole milk, cream, sugar, chocolate chips, cocoa powder, and vanilla. Cover and cook on low for 2 hours, until the hot chocolate is hot but not boiling.

2. Turn off the slow cooker. Top with a light sprinkling of powdered sugar, salt, or cocoa powder. Serve the hot chocolate warm.

3. Refrigerate leftovers for up to 5 days.

> **TIP**
>
> If you are sensitive to chocolate and caffeine during your liquids phase of recovery, replace the chocolate chips with carob chips (1:1 ratio).

> **SERVING RECOMMENDATIONS**
>
> **Liquids:** ¼–½ cup
> **Pureed Foods:** ¼–½ cup
> **Soft Foods:** ½ cup
> **General Foods:** 1 cup

Per serving: Calories: 264; Protein: 8g; Fat: 15g; Carbohydrates: 24g; Fiber: 2g; Sugar: 22g; Sodium: 110mg

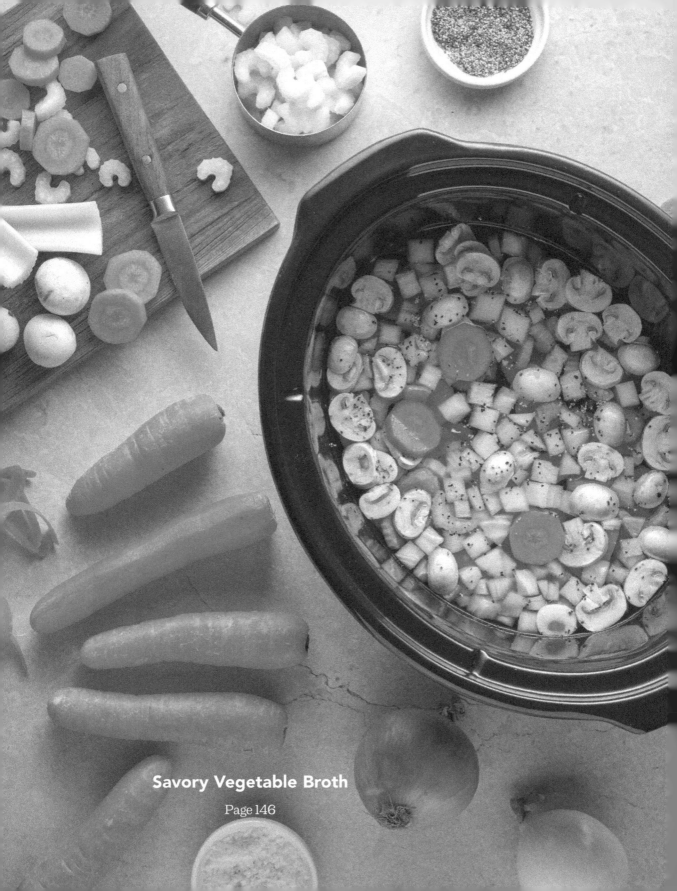

Savory Vegetable Broth

Page 146

8

Basics

Ⓛ LIQUIDS Ⓢ SOFT FOODS   PUREED FOODS Ⓖ GENERAL FOODS FOR LIFE

L P S G

Savory Chicken Broth

Prep time: 10 minutes
Cook time: 8 to 10 hours on low
SERVES 6

This warm, savory broth is delicious on its own or used as a base for many meat and poultry recipes throughout this cookbook. Perfect for your liquids phase of recovery, you can sip it warm throughout the day to stay hydrated. Or add chicken meat back into the broth for a protein-rich soup during the soft-foods phase.

3 pounds bone-in chicken pieces (like wings and thighs)

4 large carrots, sliced

1 cup chopped celery

1 medium yellow onion, diced

2 teaspoons minced garlic

1 teaspoon dried thyme

1 teaspoon dried parsley

1 teaspoon dried oregano

1 teaspoon dried rosemary

2 teaspoons sea salt

1 teaspoon ground black pepper

6 cups water

1. In a 6-quart slow cooker, combine the chicken, carrots, celery, onion, garlic, thyme, parsley, oregano, rosemary, salt, black pepper, and water. Cover and cook on low for 8 to 10 hours, until heated through.

2. Turn off the slow cooker. Strain the solids over a heat-safe container and discard the vegetables.

3. If desired, pull the chicken meat off the bones and add back to the broth for more protein (in the soft-foods and general-foods stages).

4. Serve the broth warm, or use it in other recipes.

5. Refrigerate leftovers for up to 2 weeks, or freeze for up to 3 months.

MAKE IT A MEAL

Use this broth as a base in seafood, poultry, and meat dishes, such as Easy Chicken and Rice (page 98), BBQ Pulled Pork (page 119), and Moroccan-Inspired Lamb Shanks (page 124).

If not using the chicken meat in the broth, save it to use in other soups and chilis for more protein.

Liquids: ¼–½ cup
Pureed Foods: ¼–½ cup
Soft Foods: ½ cup
General Foods: 1 cup

Per serving: Calories: 15; Protein: 2g; Fat: 0g; Carbohydrates: 2g; Fiber: 0g; Sugar: 1g; Sodium: 428mg

L P S G

Savory Vegetable Broth

Prep time: 10 minutes
Cook time: 8 to 10 hours on low
SERVES 6

This recipe is a perfect substitute for chicken broth if you are looking for a vegan or vegetarian alternative. You can use it in place of chicken broth in any recipe in this cookbook, and you can also serve it warm on its own. Perfect for your liquids recovery phase, it will help you stay hydrated while soothing your healing stomach.

8 large carrots, sliced

2 cups chopped celery

2 medium yellow onions, diced

2 cups sliced cremini mushrooms

2 teaspoons sea salt

1 teaspoon ground black pepper

6 cups water

1. In a 6-quart slow cooker, combine the carrots, celery, onions, mushrooms, salt, black pepper, and water. Cover and cook on low for 8 to 10 hours, until heated through.

2. Turn off the slow cooker. Strain the vegetables over a separate container and discard them.

3. Serve the broth warm, or use it in other recipes.

4. Refrigerate leftovers for up to 2 weeks, or freeze for up to 3 months.

MAKE IT A MEAL

Use this broth as a base in vegetarian and seafood recipes, or add protein by throwing in 2 ounces of edamame or cooked lentils after cooking.

SERVING RECOMMENDATIONS

Liquids: ¼–½ cup
Pureed Foods: ¼–½ cup
Soft Foods: ½ cup
General Foods: 1 cup

Per serving: Calories: 10; Protein: 0g; Fat: 0g; Carbohydrates: 3g; Fiber: 0g; Sugar: 3g; Sodium: 388mg

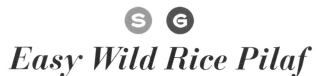

Easy Wild Rice Pilaf

Prep time: 10 minutes
Cook time: 6 to 8 hours on low, plus 10 minutes to rest
SERVES 6

"Easy and delicious" is how I describe this whole-grain side dish! Wild rice provides essential fiber and minerals for a nutrition powerhouse side dish. It's also bursting with flavor from the broth, mushrooms, onion, and thyme. It's perfect for your soft-foods phase of recovery, as a side dish or on its own if you need something simple.

3 tablespoons extra-virgin olive oil, divided

2 cups wild rice, rinsed and drained

1 medium white onion, diced

1¼ cups sliced cremini mushrooms

4 cups Savory Chicken Broth (page 144) or store-bought chicken broth

½ teaspoon sea salt

½ teaspoon ground black pepper

1 teaspoon dried thyme

1. Coat the bottom and sides of a 6-quart slow cooker with 1 tablespoon of olive oil.

2. Add the rice, onion, mushrooms, broth, salt, black pepper, and thyme. Cover and cook on low for 6 to 8 hours, until all the liquid has been absorbed by the rice.

3. Turn off the slow cooker. Remove the lid and stir in the remaining 2 tablespoons of olive oil. Replace the lid and let the rice sit for 10 minutes.

4. Serve the pilaf warm or as a side dish with other recipes.

5. Refrigerate leftovers for up to 1 week, or freeze for up to 3 months.

MAKE IT A MEAL

Serve with any seafood or poultry dish, such as Creole Chicken and Sausage (page 120) or Easy Seafood Stew (page 70), or use as a base with chili.

SERVING RECOMMENDATIONS

Soft Foods: ¼ cup
General Foods: ¼–½ cup

Per serving: Calories: 261; Protein: 8g; Fat: 7g; Carbohydrates: 42g; Fiber: 4g; Sugar: 2g; Sodium: 102mg

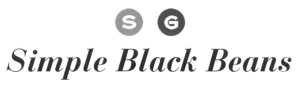

Simple Black Beans

Prep time: 5 minutes
Cook time: 6 to 8 hours on low
SERVES 10 TO 12

Black beans go with so many other dishes! Definitely keep these on hand to quickly add protein and fiber to almost any meal. The simple savory flavor of these black beans means they go well in tacos, in casseroles, as salad toppings, and as a side dish. They are also gentle on your healing stomach, perfect for your soft-foods phase.

1 pound dried black beans, rinsed (not soaked)

⅛ teaspoon garlic powder

2 teaspoons onion powder

1 tablespoon sea salt

¼ cup extra-virgin olive oil

8 cups Savory Chicken Broth (page 144), Savory Vegetable Broth (page 146), or store-bought broth

1. In a 6-quart slow cooker, combine the beans, garlic powder, onion powder, salt, and olive oil.

2. Pour the broth over the beans and spices. Cover and cook on low for 6 to 8 hours, until the beans are very soft and most of the liquid has been absorbed.

3. Turn off the slow cooker. Serve the beans warm or use in other recipes.

4. Refrigerate leftovers (in their cooking liquid to retain moisture) for up to 1 week, or freeze for up to 3 months.

TIP

Start checking the doneness of the beans around 4 hours in. Slow cookers vary, and cooking times for legumes and whole grains may be less than what you plan for.

SERVING RECOMMENDATIONS

Soft Foods: ½ cup
General Foods: 1 cup

Per serving: Calories: 204; Protein: 10g; Fat: 6g; Carbohydrates: 29g; Fiber: 7g; Sugar: 1g; Sodium: 352mg

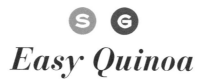

Easy Quinoa

Prep time: 5 minutes
Cook time: 5 to 6 hours on low
SERVES 8 TO 10

Boost your fiber, protein, zinc, iron, and magnesium intake with this whole grain. Easy to assemble and cook, it combines well with other dishes for flavor and depth. Quinoa is a great team player with poultry, red meat, fish, and legumes. It's also gentle on your healing stomach. Keep this whole grain on hand during your soft-foods phase.

2 cups quinoa, rinsed

4 cups Savory Chicken Broth (page 144), Savory Vegetable Broth (page 146), or store-bought broth

1 teaspoon sea salt

1. In a 6-quart slow cooker, combine the quinoa, broth, and salt. Cover and cook on low for 5 to 6 hours, until the liquid has been absorbed.

2. Turn off the slow cooker. Serve the quinoa warm on its own or as a side with meat, fish, poultry, or vegetarian dishes.

3. Refrigerate leftovers for up to 1 week, or freeze for up to 3 months.

> MAKE IT A MEAL
>
> Serve this grain with any seafood or poultry dish as a whole-grain side, or use it as a base for chili or soup. Serve it with ¼ cup of lentils or black beans for a simple meal.

SERVING RECOMMENDATIONS

Soft Foods: ½ cup
General Foods: 1 cup

Per serving: Calories: 156; Protein: 6g; Fat: 3g; Carbohydrates: 27g; Fiber: 3g; Sugar: 0g; Sodium: 147mg

Classic Bolognese Sauce

Prep time: 15 minutes
Cook time: 15 minutes on high and 6 hours on low
SERVES 10 TO 12

Bolognese sauce can be a great way to boost your protein, B vitamin, and iron intake without going to all the effort of making a main protein dish, thanks to the generous amount of ground beef. Additionally, the vegetables boost antioxidants and fiber, making this a gentle, digestion-friendly pasta sauce during your soft-foods phase.

2 tablespoons extra-virgin olive oil

4 teaspoons minced garlic

1 medium yellow onion, finely chopped

½ cup finely diced celery

½ cup finely diced carrots

2 teaspoons sea salt, divided

½ teaspoon ground black pepper

2 pounds 85- or 90-percent lean ground beef

1 tablespoon dried oregano

2 teaspoons dried thyme

1 teaspoon cayenne pepper

1 cup red wine (preferably cabernet sauvignon or merlot)

3 tablespoons tomato paste

2 (28-ounce) cans crushed tomatoes

1 cup 2 percent milk

1. Coat the bottom and sides of a 6-quart slow cooker with the olive oil.

2. Set the heat to high. Add the garlic and onion. Cook, stirring occasionally, for 4 to 5 minutes, until fragrant.

3. Stir in the celery and carrots. Cook for 3 to 4 minutes.

4. Add the salt, black pepper, beef, oregano, thyme, cayenne, and wine. Mix well. Cook for 5 minutes, until most, if not all, of the wine evaporates.

5. Stir in the tomato paste and crushed tomatoes. Cover, reduce the heat to low, and cook for 5 hours, until the sauce has thickened.

6. Remove the lid and mix in the milk. Replace the lid and cook for an additional 1 hour.

7. Turn off the slow cooker. Serve the Bolognese warm as a sauce for pasta, vegetables, or potatoes or use in lasagna.

8. Refrigerate leftovers for up to 5 days, or freeze for up to 3 months.

MAKE IT A MEAL

Serve over ¼ to ½ cup of cooked whole-grain or gluten-free pasta and top with 2 tablespoons of Parmesan cheese.

SERVING RECOMMENDATIONS

Soft Foods: ½ cup
General Foods: 1 cup

Per serving: Calories: 256; Protein: 21g; Fat: 13g; Carbohydrates: 11g; Fiber: 4g; Sugar: 6g; Sodium: 499mg

S **G**

Versatile Baked Potatoes

Prep time: 5 minutes
Cook time: 6 to 8 hours on low
SERVES 10 TO 12

A baked potato is one of my favorite comfort foods because you can top it with just about anything: chili, cheese, Bolognese sauce, sour cream, chives, onions, fajita mix, salsa, butter, olive oil, or eggs. Save these versatile potatoes for quick and easy comfort meals. Since these potatoes are very soft in the center, they are perfect for your soft-foods phase.

1 tablespoon extra-virgin olive oil

1 teaspoon sea salt

1 teaspoon ground black pepper

6 medium russet potatoes, washed

1¼ to 1½ cups olive oil, butter, sour cream, shredded cheese, or Bolognese sauce (optional)

1. In a small bowl, combine the olive oil, sea salt, and black pepper.

2. Rub the olive oil mixture thoroughly over each potato. Pierce each potato 8 or 10 times using a fork.

3. Arrange the potatoes in the slow cooker. Cover and cook on low for 6 to 8 hours, until the potatoes are soft and fork tender.

4. Turn off the slow cooker. Cut open each potato and top with 2 tablespoons of olive oil, butter, sour cream, shredded cheese, or Bolognese sauce per serving (if using). Serve the potatoes warm.

5. Refrigerate leftovers for up to 5 days, or freeze for up to 3 months.

MAKE IT A MEAL

Top with ¼ cup of Classic Bolognese Sauce (page 150) or chili and shredded cheese for protein, or serve as a side with any poultry, seafood, or meat dish.

SERVING RECOMMENDATIONS

Soft Foods: ½ cup
General Foods: 1 cup

Per serving: Calories: 113; Protein: 3g; Fat: 1g; Carbohydrates: 23g; Fiber: 2g; Sugar: 1g; Sodium: 123mg

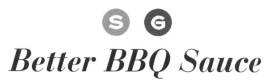

Better BBQ Sauce

Prep time: 5 minutes
Cook time: 6 to 8 hours on low
SERVES 10 TO 12

Natural sweeteners make this a better BBQ sauce. Most store-bought varieties contain corn syrup for sweetener, but I use coconut sugar and honey instead. You can also use molasses and maple syrup if you wish. Enjoy this sweet and tangy sauce on your protein of choice during your soft-foods phase.

1 (28-ounce) can tomato puree

¾ cup coconut sugar

2 teaspoons onion powder

¼ cup apple cider vinegar

¼ cup honey

2 teaspoons whiskey (optional)

1 tablespoon chili powder

1 tablespoon yellow mustard

2 teaspoons liquid smoke

¼ teaspoon garlic powder

1 teaspoon sea salt

1 teaspoon ground black pepper

1. In a 6-quart slow cooker, combine the tomato puree, sugar, onion powder, vinegar, honey, whiskey (if using), chili powder, mustard, liquid smoke, garlic powder, salt, and black pepper. Cover and cook on low for 6 to 8 hours, until the sauce has thickened (for a thicker sauce, leave the lid cracked a little bit, especially for the last couple of hours).

2. Turn off the slow cooker. Spoon the sauce into glass containers to store. Let cool to room temperature before refrigerating.

3. Refrigerate leftovers for up to 2 weeks, or freeze for up to 3 months.

MAKE IT A MEAL

Combine with 2 ounces of pulled chicken, beef, or pork for sandwiches, or use as a sauce over any protein and serve with ¼ cup of a vegetable side.

SERVING RECOMMENDATIONS

Soft Foods: ¼ cup
General Foods: ¼ cup

Per serving: Calories: 126; Protein: 2g; Fat: 0g; Carbohydrates: 31g; Fiber: 2g; Sugar: 26g; Sodium: 182mg

Homemade Alfredo Sauce

Prep time: 15 minutes
Cook time: 5 minutes on high and 2 hours 30 minutes on low
SERVES 8 TO 10

Benefits of making your own Alfredo sauce? Fresher flavor and fewer preservatives! This creamy sauce is an excellent topping for pasta and protein alike. Make it in large batches, and save it for future meals when you need to warm up a sauce quickly. It can also bring plain chicken or fish alive for a more satisfying meal.

2 tablespoons extra-virgin olive oil

½ teaspoon minced garlic

2 tablespoons butter

3 tablespoons whole-wheat flour, plus more as needed

1 teaspoon garlic powder

2 cups 2 percent milk

¾ cup heavy (whipping) cream

¾ cup water

⅓ cup shredded white Cheddar cheese

1 cup grated Parmesan cheese

½ teaspoon sea salt

Ground black pepper

1. In a 6-quart slow cooker, combine the olive oil and garlic. Cook on high, stirring frequently, for 3 to 4 minutes, until fragrant.

2. Add the butter and stir until melted.

3. Whisk in the flour until well combined.

4. Stir in the garlic powder, milk, cream, and water. Cover, reduce the heat to low, and cook for 2 hours.

5. Remove the lid and stir in the Cheddar cheese, Parmesan cheese, salt, and black pepper.

6. Replace the lid and cook for an additional 20 to 30 minutes, until the cheese has melted and the sauce is thick and creamy. (If the sauce has not thickened to your liking, add another 1 to 2 teaspoons of flour until the desired consistency is reached.)

7. Turn off the slow cooker. Serve the sauce warm over whole-grain or gluten-free pasta or a protein of your choice. Spoon leftover sauce into glass containers. Let cool to room temperature before refrigerating.

8. Refrigerate leftovers for up to 4 days, or freeze for up to 2 months.

Serve over ¼ cup of cooked whole-grain or gluten-free pasta, and include 1 to 2 ounces of a protein of your choice (chicken or fish for best flavor).

SERVING RECOMMENDATIONS

Soft Foods: ½ cup
General Foods: 1 cup

Per serving: Calories: 245; Protein: 8g; Fat: 21g; Carbohydrates: 8g; Fiber: 0g; Sugar: 4g; Sodium: 389mg

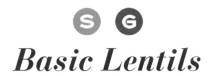

Basic Lentils

Prep time: 5 minutes
Cook time: 6 to 8 hours on low
SERVES 5 TO 6

Lentils are protein- and fiber-rich legumes that are also gentle on a healing stomach. They combine well with a variety of grains and starches for a complete meal, and they also provide zinc, magnesium, iron, and B vitamins. Make a large batch ahead, as they are easy to warm up when you need a quick meal or side.

1 cup dried brown or green lentils, rinsed

7 cups water

Sea salt

Ground black pepper

1. In a 6-quart slow cooker, combine the lentils and water. Cover and cook on low for 6 to 8 hours, until the lentils are soft and tender and some of the liquid has been absorbed.

2. Turn off the slow cooker. Discard the excess liquid.

3. Spoon the lentils into a separate container. Season with salt and black pepper. Let cool to room temperature.

4. Refrigerate leftovers for up to 1 week, or freeze for up to 3 months.

MAKE IT A MEAL

Serve over ¼ cup of cooked whole-grain or gluten-free pasta, rice, or cauliflower rice, or serve as a side with 1 to 2 ounces of protein and ¼ cup of a vegetable of your choice.

SERVING RECOMMENDATIONS

Soft Foods: ½ cup
General Foods: 1 cup

Per serving: Calories: 135; Protein: 9g; Fat: 0g; Carbohydrates: 24g; Fiber: 4g; Sugar: 1g; Sodium: 10mg

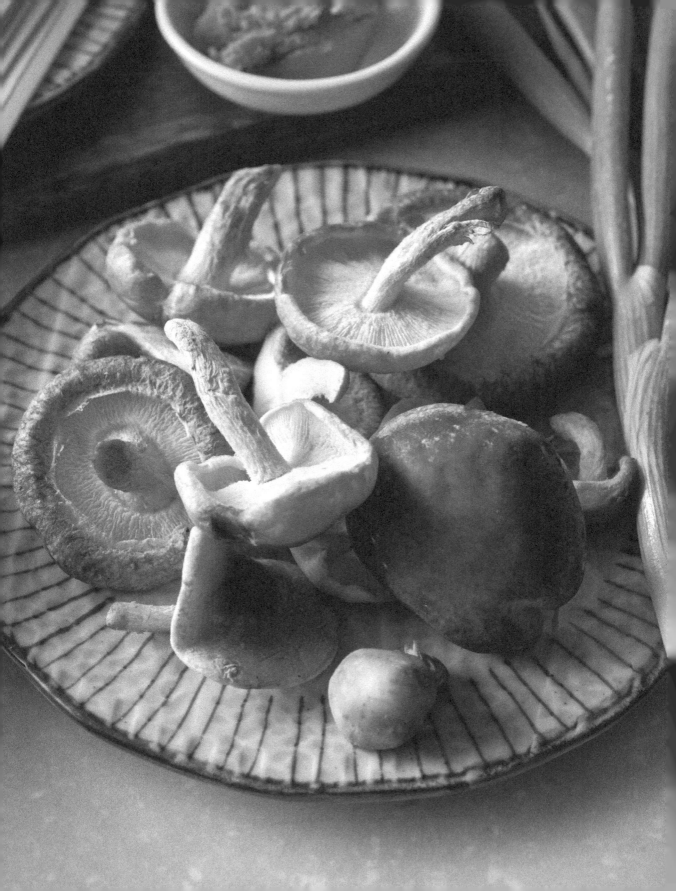

MEASUREMENT CONVERSIONS

	US STANDARD	US STANDARD (OUNCES)	METRIC (APPROXIMATE)
VOLUME EQUIVALENTS (LIQUID)	2 TABLESPOONS	1 FL. OZ.	30 ML
	¼ CUP	2 FL. OZ.	60 ML
	½ CUP	4 FL. OZ.	120 ML
	1 CUP	8 FL. OZ.	240 ML
	1½ CUPS	12 FL. OZ.	355 ML
	2 CUPS OR 1 PINT	16 FL. OZ.	475 ML
	4 CUPS OR 1 QUART	32 FL. OZ.	1 L
	1 GALLON	128 FL. OZ.	4 L
VOLUME EQUIVALENTS (DRY)	⅛ TEASPOON		0.5 ML
	¼ TEASPOON		1 ML
	½ TEASPOON		2 ML
	¾ TEASPOON		4 ML
	1 TEASPOON		5 ML
	1 TABLESPOON		15 ML
	¼ CUP		59 ML
	⅓ CUP		79 ML
	½ CUP		118 ML
	⅔ CUP		156 ML
	¾ CUP		177 ML
	1 CUP		235 ML
	2 CUPS OR 1 PINT		475 ML
	3 CUPS		700 ML
	4 CUPS OR 1 QUART		1 L
	½ GALLON		2 L
	1 GALLON		4 L

OVEN TEMPERATURES

FAHRENHEIT	CELSIUS (APPROXIMATE)
250°F	120°C
300°F	150°C
325°F	165°C
350°F	180°C
375°F	190°C
400°F	200°C
425°F	220°C
450°F	230°C

WEIGHT EQUIVALENTS

U.S. STANDARD	METRIC (APPROXIMATE)
½ OUNCE	15 G
1 OUNCE	30 G
2 OUNCES	60 G
4 OUNCES	115 G
8 OUNCES	225 G
12 OUNCES	340 G
16 OUNCES OR 1 POUND	455 G

REFERENCES

Foster, Kelli. "The Easy Way to Adapt Recipes to the Size of Your Slow Cooker."
The Kitchn (blog). Last modified May 1, 2019. TheKitchn.com/the-easy-way-to
-adapt-recipes-for-large-and-small-slow-cookers-228510.

Mayo Clinic. "Gastric Bypass Diet: What to Eat After the Surgery." Accessed
September 25, 2021. MayoClinic.org/tests-procedures/gastric-bypass-surgery
/in-depth/gastric-bypass-diet/art-20048472.

NutritionFacts.org. Accessed September 26, 2021. NutritionFacts.org.

Penn Medicine. "What Foods and Drinks Should You Avoid after Bariatric Surgery?"
January 5, 2020. PennMedicine.org/updates/blogs/metabolic-and-bariatric-surgery
-blog/2020/january/foods-drinks-to-avoid-after-bariatric-surgery.

Phoenix Health. "Eight Foods to Avoid after Bariatric Surgery." Accessed September 26,
2021. Phoenix-Health.co.uk/foods-to-avoid-after-bariatric-surgery.

Recipes that Crock! "How to Adjust Crock Pot Servings." Accessed
September 26, 2021. RecipesthatCrock.com/resourcestips-tools/how-to
-adjust-crock-pot-servings.

UCSF Health. "Dietary Guidelines after Bariatric Surgery." Accessed September 23,
2021. UCSFHealth.org/education/dietary-guidelines-after-bariatric-surgery.

UPMC. "Clear Liquid Diet for Post-Bariatric and Weight Loss Surgery Patients." Accessed
September 24, 2021. UPMC.com/services/bariatrics/surgery-process/post-surgery
/diet/clear-liquid.

UPMC. "Full Liquid Diet for Bariatric Gastric Band Post-Surgery Patients." Accessed September 24, 2021. UPMC.com/services/bariatrics/surgery-process/post-surgery /diet/full-liquid.

UPMC. "Phase 2B: Pureed Food Diet for Post-Bariatric Surgery Patients." Accessed September 24, 2021. UPMC.com/services/bariatrics/surgery-process/post-surgery /diet/pureed.

UPMC. "Phase 3: Adaptive or Soft Food Diet for Post-Bariatric Surgery Patients." Accessed September 24, 2021. UPMC.com/services/bariatrics/surgery-process/post -surgery/diet/soft.

UPMC. "Phase 4: Stabilization Diet for Post-Bariatric Surgery Patients." Accessed September 25, 2021. UPMC.com/services/bariatrics/surgery-process/post-surgery /diet/stabilization.

UPMC. "Post Bariatric Surgery Diet." Accessed September 25, 2021. UPMC.com/services /bariatrics/surgery-process/post-surgery/diet.

Vito, Victoria. "Why Is Slow Cooking Good For You?" *HuffPost UK*. Last modified November 24, 2017. HuffingtonPost.co.uk/victoria-vito/why-is-slow-cooking -good-_b_13184760.html.

Whelan, Corey. "Gastric Sleeve Diet." *Healthline*. Last modified July 2, 2019. Healthline.com/health/gastric-sleeve-diet.

INDEX

ACKNOWLEDGMENTS

Thank you to the Callisto team for being precise and supportive in their recommendations and process. It takes a village!

ABOUT THE AUTHOR

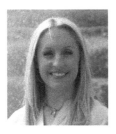 **Lauren Minchen** is a registered dietitian nutritionist. At her nutrition practice, Lauren Minchen Nutrition, she specializes in digestive health and autoimmune conditions. She lives in New York City with her husband and son.